Prevention of Dementia

The Art and Science of Sustaining Cognitive Well-Being

Rafael Dias

First edition

Contents

I

Part One

Introduction to the Book

U nveiling the Marvels of the Mind!

Imagine your brain as a fantastic supercomputer nestled within your skull. This book serves as your map, guiding you through the inner workings of this remarkable machine and revealing ways to enhance its capabilities.

What Awaits You?

Prepare for an exploration into different facets of brain health. From understanding early signs of challenges to adopting habits that nourish your brain, each chapter is like a puzzle piece that contributes to the larger picture of a healthy and active mind.

The Relevance

Just as superheroes train to harness their powers, our brains need specialized care. This book is your Brain Training Camp, offering insights and strategies to optimize memory, cognitive function, and overall mental well-being.

Are you ready for this adventure? Let's venture into the world of brain health together and unlock the secrets that lie within!

About the Author: A Lifelong Quest for Truth in Cognitive Health

My journey has been a relentless pursuit of truth, a quest that has spanned a lifetime. From the very outset, I embarked on this expedition not merely as an observer but as a fervent seeker of knowledge, determined to decipher the mysteries of the mind and uncover groundbreaking solutions to one of humanity's most formidable challenges — dementia.

The Early Days of Inquiry

From the earliest days of my academic pursuits, I felt a burning curiosity to understand the intricacies of the human brain. The quest for knowledge became an insatiable thirst, propelling me to delve into the most profound realms of neuroscience and cognitive science. It was during these formative years that the seeds of my lifelong commitment to unraveling the mysteries of cognitive decline were sown.

Engaging with the Best Minds

In my pursuit of truth, I have been fortunate to engage with the most brilliant minds in the field of cognitive health. Conversations with these luminaries have not only expanded my understanding but have fueled an unyielding determination to seek new and better ways to address the challenges posed by dementia. The insights gleaned from these interactions have been invaluable, shaping my perspective and propelling me forward on this unwavering journey.

A Personal Commitment

My commitment to this cause is deeply personal. I have witnessed the impact of cognitive decline on individuals and their loved ones, and it has intensified my resolve to contribute meaningfully to the fight against dementia. Every discovery, every breakthrough, is not just a triumph for science but a step closer to a world where cognitive well-being is preserved for all.

Pioneering Innovation

The search for truth has led me to the forefront of innovation. It is not enough to accept the existing paradigms; my goal is to push the boundaries, challenge assumptions, and explore avenues that promise new and effective strategies in the battle against cognitive decline. It is an endeavor that requires not just knowledge but a tenacious spirit that refuses to be bound by convention.

A Call to Action

As you delve into the pages of this book, know that it is a culmination of a lifelong quest for truth. It is an invitation to join me on this journey, to explore the frontiers of cognitive health, and to embrace the possibility of a future where dementia is not just managed but conquered. Together, let us continue to seek, discover, and pioneer the path towards a world free from the shadows of cognitive decline.

Dedication

To my dearest wife, Cherene, and our two beautiful daughters, Arazona and Phoenix.

This book is dedicated to you, the pillars of my strength, the lights that illuminate my life. Your unwavering support and boundless love have been my guiding stars on this journey.

Cherene, your grace, resilience, and the warmth of your love have been my sanctuary in times of challenge. Arazona and Phoenix, your laughter, curiosity, and the joy you bring into our home inspire me daily.

May the insights within these pages reflect the gratitude I hold for each of you. Your love fuels my pursuit of knowledge, and it is in your embrace that I find the strength to navigate the complex terrain of life's endeavors.

With all my love

II

Part Two

Understanding Dementia

Introduction to Dementia

Welcome to the intricate realm of dementia, a subject that goes far beyond medical terminology and delves deep into the fabric of human experience. This chapter serves as the opening curtain to a journey of understanding, empathy, and the pursuit of knowledge regarding one of the most complex challenges faced by individuals and their loved ones.

Defining Dementia

At its core, dementia is not just a condition but a profound shift in the way individuals experience and engage with the world. It encompasses a range of cognitive impairments that affect memory, reasoning, and daily functioning. As we embark on this exploration, our aim is to unravel the layers of dementia, shedding light on its multifaceted nature.

The Human Impact

Beyond the clinical definitions, we must recognize the human impact of dementia. It transforms lives, reshaping relationships and challenging the very essence of identity. Through this exploration, we seek to understand not only the medical aspects but also the emotional and social dimensions that accompany a dementia diagnosis.

Navigating the Unknown

Dementia is often uncharted territory, a landscape filled with uncertainties and complexities. This chapter acts as a compass, guiding us through the unknown territories of cognitive decline. By navigating these intricacies, we lay the foundation for a comprehensive understanding of the challenges posed by dementia.

An Invitation to Knowledge

Our journey is not one of despair but of empowerment through knowledge. As we dive into the subsequent chapters, we will equip ourselves with insights that illuminate the origins, symptoms, and potential interventions for dementia. This exploration is an invitation to join the collective effort to demystify and confront this condition.

A Holistic Perspective

Beyond the clinical aspects, we emphasize a holistic perspective that acknowledges the individual behind the diagnosis. By recognizing the human experience of dementia, we pave the way for a more compassionate and informed approach to supporting those affected and their communities.

So, let's embark on this quest for understanding—a journey that goes beyond the medical textbooks and delves into the heart of what it means to grapple with dementia. Together, we navigate the complexities, armed with curiosity, compassion, and a shared commitment to unraveling the intricacies that surround this condition.

Types of Dementia

We're about to dive into the world of dementia, where different types of brain challenges await. It's like exploring a big puzzle, trying to understand how each piece fits in.

Alzheimer's Adventure: Memory Lane

Let's start with Alzheimer's disease, the most common type of dementia. Think of it like a journey where memory starts playing hide-and-seek, and thinking becomes a bit tricky. We'll uncover the mysteries behind Alzheimer's and what makes it unique.

Vascular Voyage: Through Blood Rivers

Next up is vascular dementia. Imagine it as a journey through the rivers in our brains. Sometimes, when these rivers get a bit tricky, it can cause problems with thinking and remembering. Let's navigate these waters together.

Lewy Body Discovery: Protein Puzzles

Now, let's uncover Lewy Body dementia. It's like solving a puzzle where proteins in the brain act a bit differently. This one brings surprises like seeing things that aren't there and changes in how alert someone is.

Frontotemporal Quest: Personality and Behavior Expedition

Ever wondered about the areas of the brain that shape personality and behavior? That's where frontotemporal dementia comes in. It's like going on an expedition to understand why someone might start acting differently or having trouble with language.

Mixed Dementia Maze: A Bit of Everything

Picture mixed dementia as a maze where more than one type of dementia joins the adventure. It's like having a combination of puzzles to solve, making things a bit more complicated.

Other Rare Challenges: Uncommon but Important

Beyond the big types, there are also rare challenges like Creutzfeldt-Jakob and Huntington's diseases. These are like rare gems, less common but still significant pieces of the puzzle.

Putting It All Together

So, our journey isn't just about one type; it's about understanding how all these different puzzles fit together. Each type is like a unique color in a big painting, showing us the rich variety within the world of dementia.

As we explore the different types of dementia, discovering what makes each one special. It's a journey full of surprises and learning, and together, we'll uncover the secrets of the brain!

The Impact of Dementia on Individuals and Society

In this chapter, we'll explore how dementia can have an impact on people and our larger community.

Meet Dementia: The Memory Mix-Up

Imagine meeting someone who has a friend called Dementia. Dementia sometimes plays tricks with memory. It's like having a forgetful friend who sometimes forgets where they put things or the names of people they know.

Challenges for Families: A Puzzle to Solve

Now, let's think about families. When someone in a family has Dementia, it's like solving a puzzle together. Families may need to help more, be patient, and find new ways to communicate. It's a bit like teamwork in figuring out the pieces of the puzzle.

Friends and Feelings: The Emotional Rollercoaster

Think about having a friend with Dementia. Sometimes they might feel sad, confused, or frustrated. It's important for friends to understand and be kind, just like when we help each other in the playground.

Community Connections: Our Big Human Family

Now, let's zoom out and think about our whole community. When more people have Dementia, it's like our big human family faces a challenge. But, just like in a family, we can support each other. We might create spaces where everyone feels included or learn more about Dementia to help friends and neighbors.

Our Shared Adventure: Learning and Growing

So, what's our mission? It's like going on an adventure to learn more about Dementia, to understand how it affects people, and to make our big human family stronger. As we explore, we'll find ways to support each other and grow together.

Ready for this journey of understanding? Let's go explore the impact of Dementia on individuals and our big, wonderful human family!

The Science Behind Cognitive Decline

How the Brain Works

In the intricate landscape of human biology, the brain stands as the orchestrator of the body's myriad functions. To comprehend the marvels of cerebral intricacy, let's delve into the fascinating world of neurobiology.

The Cerebral Epicenter: The Thinking Powerhouse

At the core of the brain's operations lies the cerebrum, a vast expanse where intricate thinking processes unfold. This region is the nexus of problem-solving, critical thinking, and the imagination, allowing us to ponder complex questions and visualize far-reaching possibilities.

Navigating the Limbic Landscape: The Realm of Emotions

Venturing into the depths of the limbic system reveals the emotional epicenter. Here, the ebb and flow of feelings are regulated, giving rise to joy, sorrow, and everything in between. This neural neighborhood plays a pivotal role in shaping our emotional landscape and responses to the world around us.

The Command Center: Brainstem Operations

The brainstem serves as the command center for vital functions, managing automatic processes such as breathing, heartbeat, and digestion. This region, often overlooked, is the unsung hero ensuring the seamless operation of essential bodily functions.

Neurons: Messengers of the Mind

Picture neurons as the heralds of thought, conducting messages throughout the brain. These specialized cells transmit information, forming intricate networks that enable communication within the brain. It's the neural symphony that allows us to move, think, and experience the world.

Electric Symphony: Brain Waves in Concert

Within this cerebral metropolis, electric waves propagate through neural networks, creating the symphony of brain activity. These waves synchronize brain cells, fostering communication and coherence essential for optimal cognitive function.

Nutrients for Thought: Brain Fuel

Contrary to physical sustenance, the brain thrives on intellectual nourishment. Engaging in stimulating activities, acquiring knowledge, and exploring new experiences are the cognitive equivalent of a gourmet feast, providing the brain with the essential nutrients it craves.

Restoration in Repose: The Importance of Sleep

Every superhero requires a period of respite, and the brain is no exception. During sleep, the brain undergoes critical processes, consolidating memories, and rejuvenating its intricate neural networks. This period of repose is indispensable for cognitive vigor and sustained functionality.

In the grand tapestry of neurological wonders, the brain stands as the architect of thought, emotion, and action. As we navigate the intricate pathways of this cerebral realm, our understanding deepens, unveiling the mysteries that make the brain the unparalleled marvel it is.

Causes and Risk Factors for Cognitive Decline

I n the complex realm of cognitive health, understanding the factors contributing to cognitive decline requires an exploration into the multifaceted interplay of biology, lifestyle, and environmental influences. Let's dissect the causes and risk factors that shape the trajectory of cognitive well-being.

Genetic Blueprint: Unraveling the Code

The foundation of cognitive health is often laid by our genetic makeup. Certain genes influence susceptibility to cognitive disorders. Exploring familial medical histories can provide insights into potential genetic predispositions, offering a glimpse into the intricate genetic code that shapes cognitive destinies.

Neurological Insults: The Impact of Brain Injuries

Traumatic brain injuries and other neurological insults can disrupt cognitive function. Whether resulting from accidents, concussions, or other head traumas, these incidents may introduce challenges to cognitive health. Understanding the correlation between brain injuries and cognitive decline is paramount in unraveling this complex relationship.

Vascular Complications: Blood Flow and Cognitive Health

The vascular system plays a crucial role in maintaining cognitive function. Conditions affecting blood flow, such as hypertension or atherosclerosis, can impede the delivery of oxygen and nutrients to the brain. Exploring the intricate connection between vascular health and cognitive decline unveils a crucial aspect of the multifaceted puzzle.

Lifestyle Choices: The Impact of Habits

Our daily choices significantly influence cognitive health. Lifestyle factors such as diet, exercise, and sleep patterns play pivotal roles. A diet rich in antioxidants and omega-3 fatty acids, coupled with regular physical activity, fosters an environment conducive to cognitive well-being. Conversely, sedentary lifestyles, poor nutrition, and inadequate sleep may contribute to cognitive decline.

Environmental Exposures: Navigating External Influences

Exposure to environmental toxins and pollutants can pose challenges to cognitive health. Investigating the impact of pollutants, heavy metals, and other environmental factors provides valuable insights into potential risk factors. This exploration extends beyond personal choices, shedding light on external influences that may shape cognitive trajectories.

Psychosocial Elements: The Mind-Body Connection

The intricate connection between mental and physical health is a key consideration in understanding cognitive decline. Chronic stress, depression, and social isolation can contribute to cognitive challenges. Exploring the mind-body relationship offers valuable perspectives on the psychosocial dimensions of cognitive well-being.

Age as a Factor: Unraveling the Aging Process

As we navigate the causes of cognitive decline, the aging process emerges as a significant factor. While aging itself is not synonymous with cognitive decline, the risk of developing conditions such as Alzheimer's increases with age. Investigating the nuances of age-related cognitive changes provides a comprehensive view of the challenges associated with growing older.

In dissecting the causes and risk factors for cognitive decline, our exploration delves into the intricate interplay of genetic, environmental, and lifestyle elements. It is through understanding these multifaceted dynamics that we gain insight into the complex landscape of cognitive health.

Neurological Processes Involved in Dementia

A s we delve into the intricate realm of dementia, our exploration takes us into the inner workings of the brain, unraveling the neurological processes that underlie this complex condition. Understanding the intricate dance of neurons and the structural changes within the brain offers valuable insights into the mechanisms driving cognitive decline.

Neurotransmission: The Symphony of Chemical Messengers

At the heart of cognitive function lies neurotransmission—a symphony of chemical messengers orchestrating communication between neurons. In dementia, disruptions in this intricate dance occur. Neurotransmitters like acetylcholine, vital for memory and learning, may be compromised, leading to cognitive challenges.

Protein Aggregation: The Intricate Web of Misfolding

In various forms of dementia, abnormal protein aggregation becomes a hallmark. Proteins like beta-amyloid and tau misfold, forming plaques and tangles that interfere with neuronal function. This process, akin to a molecular glitch, disrupts the normal flow of information in the brain.

Neuronal Damage: The Fraying of Connections

Dementia often involves the deterioration of neuronal structures. Synapses, the connections between neurons, may weaken or be lost altogether. This neuronal damage contributes to the decline in cognitive abilities, as the pathways for communication within the brain become frayed.

Brain Atrophy: The Shrinking Landscape

An observable phenomenon in dementia is brain atrophy—a reduction in the size of certain brain regions. The hippocampus, crucial for memory, is particularly vulnerable. This shrinkage correlates with memory loss and cognitive decline, underscoring the physical impact of dementia on the brain's structure.

Inflammation: The Double-Edged Sword

Inflammatory processes play a dual role in dementia. While inflammation is a natural response to injury or infection, chronic inflammation in the brain can contribute to neurodegeneration. This delicate balance between protective and harmful inflammation adds another layer of complexity to the neurological processes at play.

Vascular Contributions: Blood Flow and Cognitive Function

Vascular factors also intertwine with neurological processes in dementia. Reduced blood flow to the brain, often associated with conditions like vascular dementia, can lead to oxygen deprivation and subsequent neuronal damage. Understanding the vascular dimensions of dementia is crucial for comprehending its diverse manifestations.

Genetic Influences: The Blueprint of Susceptibility

Genetic factors contribute significantly to the neurological landscape of dementia. In some cases, genetic mutations influence the production and processing of proteins implicated in neurodegeneration. Unraveling the genetic blueprint offers a glimpse into the intrinsic susceptibility to cognitive challenges.

As we navigate the neurological processes involved in dementia, it becomes apparent that this condition is a convergence of intricate molecular events, structural changes, and dynamic interplays within the brain. Our exploration of these processes is pivotal for unraveling the mysteries of dementia and developing targeted interventions to mitigate its impact.

Recognizing Early Signs of Cognitive Decline

Memory Loss and Forgetfulness

Memory, the intricate tapestry of recollection woven into the fabric of our consciousness, is both a marvel and, at times, a source of challenge. As we explore the realms of memory loss and forgetfulness, we delve into the complexities that underlie these phenomena, seeking to understand the nuanced interplay between cognition and the elusive nature of memory.

Memory: The Mosaic of Cognition

Memory is the cornerstone of our cognitive architecture, allowing us to store, retrieve, and utilize information. It comprises different forms, from short-term recall to long-term retention, collectively shaping our experiences and defining our sense of self.

Normal Forgetfulness: The Ephemeral Nature of Recall

In the realm of normalcy, forgetfulness is a common companion. Misplacing keys, drawing blanks on names, or forgetting minor details are ordinary manifestations. These instances, often linked to the complexities of daily life, seldom raise alarms.

Age-Related Memory Changes: Navigating Cognitive Shifts

As the chapters of life unfold, so do subtle shifts in memory. Age-related changes, such as slower recall and the occasional tip-of-the-tongue phenomenon, are part of the natural trajectory. Understanding these nuances distinguishes normal aging from potential concerns.

Mild Cognitive Impairment: The Gray Area

Mild cognitive impairment (MCI) marks a subtle departure from typical age-related changes. Individuals with MCI may experience more noticeable memory lapses, impacting daily functioning. Recognizing these shifts becomes crucial in discerning potential precursors to more severe cognitive challenges.

Dementia and Memory Decline: The Unraveling Threads

In the intricate tapestry of memory, dementia unravels threads that bind cognition together. Memory decline becomes more pronounced, with individuals grappling not only with forgetfulness but also with the distortion of time, difficulty learning new information, and challenges in problem-solving.

Alzheimer's Disease: A Profound Memory Odyssey

At the forefront of memory-related challenges stands Alzheimer's disease, where memory loss takes center stage. Short-term memory falters, and individuals may struggle to recognize close acquaintances or recall recent events. The gradual erosion of memory becomes a poignant narrative within the Alzheimer's odyssey.

Emotional Impact: The Echoes of Forgetfulness

Memory loss and forgetfulness resonate beyond the cognitive realm, echoing emotionally in the lives of individuals and their loved ones. The frustration of misplaced memories, the anguish of forgotten moments, and the gradual erosion of shared recollections cast a poignant shadow on the human experience.

Seeking Understanding: A Journey into Memory's Depths

Our exploration into memory loss and forgetfulness is a journey into the depths of cognition, where the intricacies of memory intertwine with the complexities of the mind. As we navigate this terrain, we aim to decipher the subtle nuances that distinguish normal forgetfulness from potential precursors to cognitive challenges, offering insights into the delicate balance of memory in the human experience.

Changes in Cognitive Abilities

In the labyrinth of cognitive function, the ebbs and flows of mental capacities mark the ever-evolving landscape of our intellectual prowess. As we embark on an exploration of changes in cognitive abilities, we dissect the intricate interplay of factors that shape the trajectory of our mental acuity.

Fluid Intelligence: The Stream of Adaptive Thinking

Cognitive abilities are multifaceted, with fluid intelligence representing the stream of adaptive thinking. This encompasses problem-solving, reasoning, and the ability to grasp new concepts swiftly. In the vibrant tapestry of cognitive prowess, fluid intelligence flows dynamically, adapting to novel challenges.

Crystallized Intelligence: The Reservoir of Accumulated Knowledge

In tandem with fluid intelligence, crystallized intelligence forms the reservoir of accumulated knowledge. This encompasses the wisdom amassed over time, encompassing facts, vocabulary, and cultural understanding. The interplay between fluid and crystallized intelligence crafts the mosaic of cognitive abilities.

Processing Speed: The Tempo of Thought

Processing speed dictates the tempo of thought processes. It involves how swiftly our minds can absorb and respond to information. Changes in processing speed may manifest as a subtle slowing down, influencing how efficiently we navigate mental tasks.

Working Memory: The Mental Sketchpad

Working memory, akin to a mental sketchpad, enables us to temporarily hold and manipulate information. Changes in this cognitive domain may manifest as difficulties in managing multiple pieces of information simultaneously, impacting tasks that require mental juggling.

Executive Functions: The Cognitive Command Center

Executive functions serve as the cognitive command center, overseeing processes like decision-making, planning, and goal-setting. Alterations in executive functions may result in challenges in organizing thoughts, making sound judgments, and executing complex tasks.

Attention and Concentration: The Spotlight of Cognition

Attention and concentration function as the spotlight of cognition, allowing us to focus on specific stimuli amid competing distractions. Changes in these domains may lead to difficulties in sustaining attention or quickly shifting focus, influencing our ability to engage with tasks.

Language Skills: The Verbal Symphony

Language skills orchestrate the verbal symphony of communication. Changes in this realm may manifest as difficulties in finding the right words, expressing thoughts coherently, or comprehending complex language structures.

Spatial Abilities: Navigating Mental Maps

Spatial abilities involve mental navigation, encompassing skills like orientation, spatial reasoning, and object manipulation. Changes in spatial abilities may influence our capacity to visualize objects in space or mentally manipulate shapes.

Multitasking: The Cognitive Juggling Act

Multitasking, the cognitive juggling act, involves managing multiple tasks simultaneously. Changes in this domain may result in challenges in efficiently dividing attention among various activities, impacting our ability to multitask seamlessly.

Emotional Regulation: The Intersection of Cognition and Emotion

Cognitive abilities intersect with emotional regulation, influencing how we manage and respond to emotions. Changes in this intersection may manifest as alterations in mood regulation, coping mechanisms, and the ability to navigate emotionally charged situations.

As we traverse the terrain of changes in cognitive abilities, our understanding deepens, revealing the intricate interplay of factors that shape the ebb and flow of mental acuity. This exploration is a crucial step in discerning normal cognitive fluctuations from potential precursors to more profound challenges, contributing to a comprehensive comprehension of the dynamic nature of human cognition.

Behavioral and Emotional Indicators

ehavioral and emotional indicators serve as poignant brushstrokes, revealing the nuances of the human experience. As we navigate this chapter, we unravel the subtle shifts in behavior and emotion that often herald the presence of underlying cognitive challenges.

Changes in Social Interactions: The Shifting Dynamics

One of the first canvases to reflect cognitive changes is social interaction. Individuals experiencing cognitive challenges may exhibit alterations in their ability to engage with others. Social withdrawal, difficulty in maintaining conversations, or a shift in interpersonal dynamics can signify underlying cognitive shifts.

Mood Swings and Emotional Fluctuations: The Emotional Palette

Emotional fluctuations often accompany cognitive changes. Mood swings, heightened irritability, or unexplained shifts in emotional states may serve as indicators. Understanding the emotional palette becomes essential in decoding the complex interplay between cognition and affective experiences.

Loss of Initiative and Motivation: The Fading Drive

A noticeable decline in initiative and motivation can be a telltale sign of cognitive challenges. Individuals may exhibit reduced interest in activities they once enjoyed, a lack of enthusiasm for new endeavors, or a general decline in the drive to pursue personal goals.

Changes in Personal Care: The Reflection in Self-Care

Personal care habits can mirror cognitive changes. Neglect of personal hygiene, difficulties in dressing appropriately, or lapses in grooming routines may point to underlying cognitive challenges. Observing changes in these daily rituals provides insights into the intricate intersections of cognition and self-care.

Disorientation in Time and Space: Navigating the Mental Map

Disorientation in time and space often surfaces in individuals grappling with cognitive challenges. Losing track of dates, forgetting the day of the week, or experiencing confusion about one's location can indicate disruptions in the cognitive mapping of temporal and spatial dimensions.

Difficulty with Familiar Tasks: The Challenge of Routine

Cognitive challenges may manifest in the struggle to perform familiar tasks. Difficulties in following recipes, navigating well-known routes, or completing routine chores may signal changes in cognitive abilities. These challenges underscore the intricate connection between cognition and daily functionality.

Repetitive Behaviors: The Echo of Routine

Repetitive behaviors, such as asking the same question repeatedly or performing specific actions in a ritualistic manner, can emerge as behavioral indicators. These patterns often echo an attempt to navigate cognitive uncertainties or find familiarity in a changing cognitive landscape.

Changes in Judgment: The Prism of Decision-Making

Cognitive changes may cast a prism on decision-making abilities. Individuals may exhibit impaired judgment, making choices that seem out of character or lack logical coherence. Recognizing alterations in decision-making processes is crucial in discerning potential cognitive challenges.

Agitation and Restlessness: The Unsettled State

Agitation and restlessness may surface as emotional responses to cognitive challenges. Individuals may exhibit heightened anxiety, pacing, or an inability to sit still. Understanding these manifestations sheds light on the emotional dimensions accompanying cognitive shifts.

Resistance to Change: The Unsettled Comfort Zone

A resistance to change, often rooted in an attempt to maintain a semblance of the familiar, may emerge. Individuals facing cognitive challenges may exhibit discomfort or frustration in the face of alterations to routines or environments, seeking stability in a changing cognitive landscape.

As we explore the behavioral and emotional indicators of cognitive challenges, we recognize the intricate tapestry of human experience. Each brushstroke reveals not only the complexity of cognitive shifts but also the profound impact on individual identity and interpersonal dynamics. This exploration is pivotal in fostering empathy, understanding, and informed support for those navigating the labyrinth of cognitive health.

The Role of Lifestyle in Brain Health

Nutrition and Cognitive Function

The dynamic interplay between nutrition and cognitive function, the choices we make at the dinner table become integral brushstrokes shaping the portrait of our mental well-being. This chapter delves into the profound impact of nutrition on cognitive function, unraveling the intricate relationship between the foods we consume and the cognitive prowess we wield.

Brain-Boosting Nutrients: The Fuel for Thought

Our brains thrive on a medley of nutrients, each playing a unique role in supporting cognitive function. Omega-3 fatty acids, found in fatty fish, walnuts, and flaxseeds, contribute to brain health and may enhance memory and cognitive performance. Antioxidant-rich fruits and vegetables, such as blueberries and spinach, combat oxidative stress, preserving cognitive function.

Hydration and Mental Clarity: The Water-Brain Connection

Adequate hydration serves as the foundation for mental clarity. Dehydration can impair concentration, attention, and overall cognitive performance. The water-brain connection underscores the importance of staying well-hydrated to support optimal cognitive function.

Balanced Diet: The Symphony of Nutritional Harmony

A balanced diet, rich in a variety of nutrients, orchestrates the symphony of nutritional harmony essential for cognitive well-being. The Mediterranean diet, renowned for its emphasis on fruits, vegetables, whole grains, and healthy fats, emerges as a stellar example, associated with cognitive benefits and a reduced risk of cognitive decline.

Blood Sugar Balance: Nourishing Cognitive Stability

The ebb and flow of blood sugar levels profoundly impact cognitive stability. Consuming complex carbohydrates, such as whole grains, promotes sustained energy release, supporting consistent cognitive performance. Balanced meals that include proteins, fats, and carbohydrates contribute to stable blood sugar levels.

The Gut-Brain Connection: Microbiota and Mind

The gut-brain connection unveils the intricate relationship between our digestive system and cognitive function. A flourishing gut microbiota, nurtured by a diet rich in fiber and fermented foods, may positively influence cognitive health. Probiotics, found in yogurt and other fermented foods, contribute to a thriving gut ecosystem with potential cognitive benefits.

Vitamins and Minerals: Micronutrients for Mindfulness

Vitamins and minerals serve as micronutrients that play pivotal roles in cognitive function. Vitamin B complex, found in whole grains and leafy greens, supports nerve function. Minerals like iron and zinc contribute to oxygen transport and neurotransmitter synthesis, essential for optimal cognitive performance.

Cafleine and Cognitive Alertness: The Stimulant Symphony

Caffeine, a natural stimulant found in coffee and tea, has been associated with improved cognitive alertness and focus. Moderate caffeine intake can enhance short-term memory and reaction time, showcasing the stimulant symphony that contributes to cognitive benefits.

Antioxidant-Rich Teas: Sipping Cognitive Elixirs

Teas, particularly green tea, boast antioxidant-rich compounds that may offer cognitive benefits. The combination of caffeine and L-theanine, an amino acid found in tea, has been linked to improved attention and memory, highlighting the potential cognitive elixirs within our teacups.

Mindful Eating: The Art of Cognitive Savoring

Mindful eating transcends the nutritional content of our meals, emphasizing the awareness and appreciation of each bite. The practice encourages a holistic approach to nutrition, fostering a deeper connection between our dietary choices and cognitive well-being.

In navigating the intricate relationship between nutrition and cognitive function, we uncover the power of our dietary choices in sculpting the contours of mental acuity. As we embark on this exploration, let us recognize the profound impact of the foods we consume, not just on our physical well-being but on the intricate machinery of cognition that propels us through the tapestry of life.

Physical Exercise and Mental Health

This chapter unravels the profound connection between physical activity and mental health, exploring the transformative impact of movement on our cognitive landscape.

Endorphins and the Exercise High: The Feel-Good Symphony

Physical exercise ignites a symphony of endorphins, our body's natural mood lifters. These neurotransmitters create a euphoric sensation known as the exercise high, alleviating stress, anxiety, and boosting overall mood. The feel-good symphony unfolds with each step, jump, or stretch.

Brain-Derived Neurotrophic Factor (BDNF): Nourishing the Brain Garden

Exercise serves as a nutrient for the brain, fostering the release of Brain-Derived Neurotrophic Factor (BDNF). BDNF acts like a fertilizer for our neural garden, promoting the growth, survival, and connectivity of neurons. This process is vital for cognitive health, contributing to improved learning and memory.

Stress Reduction and Cortisol Regulation: The Calming Cadence

Physical exercise acts as a potent stress buster, regulating the release of cortisol, our stress hormone. Engaging in regular exercise helps establish a calming cadence, mitigating the physiological effects of stress and promoting emotional well-being.

Improved Sleep Quality: The Restorative Pillow of Activity

The relationship between physical exercise and improved sleep quality is a symbiotic one. Regular activity enhances the quality of sleep, ensuring a more restorative and rejuvenating rest. Adequate sleep, in turn, contributes to enhanced cognitive function and emotional resilience.

Enhanced Cognitive Function: The Aerobic Brain Boost

Aerobic exercise, characterized by sustained, rhythmic activities like jogging, swimming, or cycling, has been linked to enhanced cognitive function. The increased blood flow and oxygen delivery to the brain during aerobic exercise contribute to improved attention, memory, and overall cognitive performance.

Neurogenesis and Synaptic Plasticity: The Dynamic Brain Dance

Exercise sparks neurogenesis, the creation of new neurons, particularly in the hippocampus—a region crucial for learning and memory. Simultaneously, synaptic plasticity, the adaptability of existing neural connections, is enhanced. This dynamic brain dance fosters cognitive flexibility and resilience.

Social Interaction and Mental Well-being: The Community Connection

Engaging in group or team-based physical activities fosters social interaction, weaving a supportive fabric for mental well-being. The camaraderie, shared goals, and sense of belonging contribute to emotional resilience, combating feelings of isolation and loneliness.

Mind-Body Connection: Yoga and Mindfulness

Practices like yoga embody the intricate mind-body connection. Combining physical movement with mindfulness, yoga promotes mental clarity, stress reduction, and emotional balance. The meditative aspects of these practices contribute to a holistic approach to mental well-being.

Consistency and Routine: The Habitual Harmony

Establishing a consistent exercise routine creates habitual harmony, weaving physical activity into the fabric of daily life. Consistency is key in reaping the long-term cognitive and mental health benefits of exercise, transforming it from an occasional activity into a lifestyle.

Adolescence and Physical Activity: Shaping Cognitive Foundations

For young minds navigating the challenges of adolescence, physical activity plays a pivotal role in shaping cognitive foundations. Regular exercise not only contributes to physical health but also supports cognitive development, emotional resilience, and academic performance.

As we traverse the symbiotic relationship between physical exercise and mental health, let us recognize the transformative power embedded in the simple act of movement. Whether through the rhythmic beats of a jog, the meditative flow of yoga, or the camaraderie of team sports, physical activity emerges as a potent brushstroke in the masterpiece of our holistic well-being.

Sleep and Its Impact on Brain Function

T hink of sleep like the director of a big play in your life. It's not the star on the stage, but it quietly works behind the scenes to make sure everything runs smoothly for your brain. This chapter is like opening a treasure chest to discover why sleep is so important. We'll find out how it helps our brain and learn about the special connection between rest and how well our brain works.

Sleep Architecture: The Stage for Cognitive Rehearsal

Sleep unfolds in stages, each playing a unique role in cognitive rehearsal. The two main types are Rapid Eye Movement (REM) and Non-Rapid Eye Movement (NREM) sleep. NREM sleep, with its deep and light stages, sets the stage for physical restoration and memory consolidation. REM sleep, resembling a cognitive rehearsal, is where dreams unfold, and emotional processing takes center stage.

Memory Consolidation: The Nightly Archive

During the deep stages of sleep, memory consolidation occurs. It's as if the brain acts as a diligent archivist, organizing and storing the day's experiences into the memory banks.

This process strengthens neural connections and enhances the retention of information, contributing to optimal cognitive performance.

Brain Detoxification: The Silent Janitor

While we sleep, the glymphatic system—a network of vessels in the brain—becomes more active. It functions as a silent janitor, clearing away waste products that accumulate during waking hours. This detoxification process is crucial for maintaining a healthy cognitive environment and preventing the buildup of potentially harmful substances.

Hormonal Regulation: The Overnight Symphony

Sleep plays a vital role in hormonal regulation, influencing the release of growth hormone, cortisol, and melatonin. Growth hormone contributes to physical growth and repair, cortisol follows a natural circadian rhythm, and melatonin helps regulate the sleep-wake cycle. The overnight symphony of hormonal activity supports overall health and cognitive well-being.

Emotional Resilience: Navigating the Dreamscapes

Dreams that unfold during REM sleep serve as a canvas for emotional processing. It's as if the mind navigates through dreamscapes, processing and integrating emotions from daily experiences. Adequate REM sleep contributes to emotional resilience, fostering a balanced and adaptive response to life's challenges.

Sleep Deprivation: The Disrupted Performance

Conversely, sleep deprivation acts as a disruptive force in the theater of cognitive function. It impairs attention, memory, and decision-making abilities. The cognitive repercussions of insufficient sleep echo in the form of decreased alertness, reduced creativity, and compromised problem-solving skills.

Adolescent Sleep Needs: The Blueprint for Growth

During adolescence, when growth and development are at their peak, sleep needs are substantial. The recommended 8-10 hours of sleep for teenagers is crucial for physical growth, cognitive development, and emotional well-being. Adequate sleep during this period sets the blueprint for a healthy and resilient adulthood.

Sleep Hygiene: The Backstage Rituals

Ensuring quality sleep involves cultivating good sleep hygiene. This includes maintaining a consistent sleep schedule, creating a comfortable sleep environment, limiting screen time before bed, and engaging in relaxation techniques. These backstage rituals pave the way for a restful night's sleep and optimal cognitive function.

Circadian Rhythm: The Internal Clock

Our bodies operate on a circadian rhythm—a biological clock that regulates various physiological processes, including the sleep-wake cycle. Aligning daily activities with this internal clock, such as exposure to natural light during the day and dim lighting in the evening, enhances the synchronization of our circadian rhythm and promotes healthy sleep.

As we delve into the realms of sleep and its impact on brain function, let us recognize the profound role it plays in shaping our cognitive abilities, emotional resilience, and overall well-being. Just as a well-rehearsed play unfolds seamlessly on stage, the restorative power of sleep ensures that our cognitive performance takes center stage in the daily symphony of life.

Cognitive Exercises and Training

Mental Stimulation Activities

E xploring the exciting world of brain adventures! Dive into a treasure map that guides us to discover awesome activities, making our brains super clever and strong. Get ready for a journey of fun and learning, where we uncover the secrets of making our minds the coolest ever!

In the dynamic landscape of cognitive well-being, mental stimulation activities emerge as the sculptors of intellectual prowess. This chapter explores the significance of engaging our minds in various stimulating pursuits, unraveling the intricate tapestry of activities that foster cognitive agility and resilience.

Reading as a Cognitive Odyssey: The Literary Journey

Embarking on the journey of reading is akin to a cognitive odyssey. Whether delving into fiction or immersing oneself in non-fiction realms, reading engages various cognitive processes. It stimulates imagination, enhances vocabulary, and fosters critical thinking. The literary journey unfolds as a captivating exploration of the mind.

Puzzles and Brain Teasers: The Neural Gymnastics

Puzzles and brain teasers serve as the neural gymnastics of cognitive fitness. Engaging with activities like crosswords, sudoku, or logic puzzles challenges the brain, promoting problem-solving skills and pattern recognition. The mental acrobatics involved contribute to the flexibility and dexterity of cognitive function.

Learning a Musical Instrument: The Harmonic Brain Workout

Mastering a musical instrument is a harmonic brain workout. It involves the integration of motor skills, auditory processing, and memory. Learning to play an instrument stimulates multiple regions of the brain, fostering coordination and enhancing cognitive abilities. The symphony of learning becomes a melody for the mind.

Language Learning Adventures: The Linguistic Expedition

Embarking on language learning adventures is a linguistic expedition for the brain. Whether exploring a new language or deepening proficiency in an existing one, language learning engages cognitive domains associated with memory, attention, and problem-solving. The linguistic journey unfolds as a cultural and intellectual exploration.

Creative Arts Exploration: The Expressive Canvas

Engaging in creative arts, be it drawing, painting, writing, or any form of artistic expression, becomes an expressive canvas for the mind. Creative activities stimulate imagination, encourage emotional expression, and foster cognitive flexibility. The expressive canvas becomes a mirror reflecting the vibrant hues of cognitive exploration.

Critical Thinking Workouts: The Analytical Gym

Critical thinking workouts serve as the analytical gym for cognitive muscles. Engaging in activities that require evaluation, analysis, and logical reasoning sharpens cognitive skills. Whether through debates, discussions, or problem-solving exercises, these workouts enhance the ability to navigate complex intellectual terrain.

Memory Games and Mnemonics: The Recall Challenge

Memory games and mnemonic exercises become the recall challenge for the brain. These activities target memory formation and retention, honing the ability to remember information. Whether through memory card games or mnemonic devices, the recall challenge becomes a playful yet effective means of enhancing cognitive recall.

Scientific Exploration: The Inquiry Quest

Embarking on scientific exploration is an inquiry quest for the mind. Engaging with scientific concepts, conducting experiments, and exploring the wonders of the natural world stimulate curiosity and critical thinking. The inquiry quest becomes a scientific odyssey, unraveling the mysteries of the universe.

Mindfulness and Meditation: The Tranquil Retreat

Practicing mindfulness and meditation becomes a tranquil retreat for the mind. These activities, rooted in ancient traditions, foster attention, emotional regulation, and overall mental well-being. The tranquil retreat becomes a sanctuary for cultivating a calm and focused cognitive landscape.

Online Courses and Continuous Learning: The Knowledge Expedition

Participating in online courses and embracing continuous learning transforms the mind into a knowledge expedition. The accessibility of diverse educational resources allows for the exploration of new subjects, acquiring new skills, and staying intellectually engaged. The knowledge expedition becomes a perpetual journey of growth and enrichment.

The mind becomes an ever-expanding canvas, eager to absorb the vibrant hues of intellectual exploration. Each activity becomes a brushstroke, contributing to the masterpiece of cognitive agility and resilience. As we navigate the landscape of stimulating pursuits, let us recognize the transformative power they hold in shaping the contours of our intellectual journey.

Brain Training Program

brain training programs stand as modern alchemists, promising to transmute mental exercises into heightened intellectual abilities. This chapter delves into the landscape of brain training, exploring the principles, controversies, and potential benefits that define this evolving field.

Principles of Brain Training: The Cognitive Gymnasium

Brain training operates on the principles of neuroplasticity—the brain's ability to adapt and reorganize itself. These programs aim to create a cognitive gymnasium, challenging the mind with exercises designed to enhance memory, attention, problem-solving, and other cognitive functions. The premise is that consistent mental workouts can lead to measurable improvements.

Cognitive Domains Targeted: A Holistic Approach

Brain training programs target various cognitive domains, offering a holistic approach to mental fitness. Memory training focuses on enhancing recall abilities, attention exercises aim to improve focus, and problem-solving tasks seek to boost cognitive flexibility. The comprehensive nature of these programs aims to sculpt a well-rounded cognitive profile.

Controversies Surrounding Brain Training: The Skeptic's Lens

Despite their popularity, brain training programs face skepticism within the scientific community. Some studies question the transferability of skills gained in these programs to real-world scenarios. The debate centers on the extent to which improvements in specific tasks during training translate into broader cognitive enhancements in daily life.

Types of Brain Training Programs: From Apps to Workshops

Brain training comes in various forms, ranging from smartphone apps to in-person workshops. Digital platforms offer accessibility and convenience, allowing users to engage in exercises at their own pace. Workshops and programs conducted by professionals provide a structured and guided approach to cognitive enhancement.

Benefits of Brain Training: Cognitive Empowerment

Proponents argue that consistent engagement with brain training programs can yield cognitive benefits. Improved memory, increased attention span, enhanced problem-solving skills, and even potential resilience against cognitive decline in older age are among the reported advantages. The empowerment of cognitive abilities is the driving force behind the appeal of these programs.

Limitations and Caveats: The Fine Print

While some studies suggest positive outcomes, it's essential to consider the limitations and caveats associated with brain training. Individual variability in responses, the importance of task specificity, and the potential for placebo effects underscore the need for a nuanced understanding of the outcomes.

The Role of Genetics and Individual Factors: Unraveling Complexity

Genetic factors and individual differences play a role in determining the efficacy of brain training. The interplay between genetics, baseline cognitive abilities, and other individual factors contributes to the complexity of outcomes. Understanding this intricate web is crucial in gauging the potential impact of brain training on an individual level.

Integration with Lifestyle Factors: A Comprehensive Approach

Brain training is most effective when integrated into a comprehensive approach that considers lifestyle factors. Factors such as physical exercise, a balanced diet, quality sleep, and social engagement contribute to overall cognitive health. Brain training programs, when part of a holistic lifestyle, may synergistically enhance cognitive well-being.

Future Directions in Brain Training: The Evolving Frontier

As technology advances and our understanding of cognitive science deepens, the landscape of brain training continues to evolve. Virtual reality applications, adaptive algorithms, and personalized training regimens represent the frontier of innovation in this field. The future holds promise for more targeted and effective brain training interventions.

Navigating the terrain of brain training programs, we encounter a landscape where science, skepticism, and the pursuit of cognitive empowerment converge. As we explore the potential benefits and limitations, the journey unfolds as an ongoing quest to unlock the secrets of optimizing our mental capacities.

Benefits of Continuous Cognitive Engagement

Exploring the manifold benefits of consistently challenging our minds, we unravel the profound impact of lifelong learning, curiosity, and intellectual exploration on cognitive well-being.

Cognitive Resilience Across the Lifespan: The Lifelong Shield

Engaging our minds in continuous cognitive activities acts as a shield across the lifespan. Research suggests that a mentally active lifestyle may contribute to cognitive resilience, potentially reducing the risk of age-related cognitive decline and neurodegenerative conditions. Lifelong learning becomes the armor that fortifies our cognitive fortress.

Neuroplasticity in Action: Shaping the Brain's Architecture

Continuous cognitive engagement capitalizes on the principle of neuroplasticity—the brain's ability to adapt and reorganize itself. Regular mental challenges stimulate the creation of new neural connections, fostering cognitive flexibility and adaptability. It's akin to shaping the intricate architecture of our brain through the dynamic dance of learning.

Enhanced Problem-Solving Skills: The Cognitive Toolset

Consistent cognitive engagement hones our problem-solving skills, providing us with a versatile cognitive toolset. Facing diverse challenges, whether through puzzles, critical thinking exercises, or real-world problem-solving, cultivates the ability to approach problems from various angles. The cognitive toolset becomes a valuable asset in navigating the complexities of life.

Improved Memory and Learning Capacity: The Cognitive Backpack

Continuous cognitive activities contribute to an improved memory and learning capacity. Engaging with new information, acquiring new skills, and embracing novel experiences strengthen the neural pathways associated with memory and learning. The cognitive backpack becomes a reservoir of knowledge and skills, expanding with each intellectual endeavor.

Cognitive Flexibility: Adapting to Life's Variability

A mentally active lifestyle fosters cognitive flexibility—the ability to adapt to changing circumstances and think creatively. Regular exposure to diverse cognitive challenges, whether through reading, problem-solving, or learning new subjects, cultivates an openness to new ideas and an agility of thought. Cognitive flexibility becomes a compass in navigating life's variability.

Emotional Regulation and Stress Management: The Cognitive Anchor

Continuous cognitive engagement extends its influence to emotional regulation and stress management. Engaging in intellectually stimulating activities provides a cognitive anchor, promoting resilience in the face of stressors. The ability to approach challenges with a composed and adaptable mindset becomes a byproduct of consistent mental engagement.

Lifelong Learning as a Lifestyle: The Intellectual Odyssey

Adopting lifelong learning as a lifestyle transforms our existence into an intellectual odyssey. Embracing curiosity, seeking knowledge, and exploring new interests become ongoing pursuits. Lifelong learning becomes a mindset that transcends formal education, fostering a perpetual quest for intellectual enrichment.

Social Connection and Cognitive Health: The Interpersonal Tapestry

Continuous cognitive engagement often intertwines with social connection, forming an interpersonal tapestry that contributes to cognitive health. Collaborative learning, engaging in group activities, and sharing intellectual pursuits with others enhance the social dimension of cognitive well-being. The interpersonal tapestry becomes a vibrant thread in the fabric of cognitive vitality.

Quality of Life Enhancement: The Holistic Impact

The benefits of continuous cognitive engagement extend beyond the cognitive realm, influencing overall quality of life.

A mentally active lifestyle contributes to a sense of purpose, fulfillment, and satisfaction. The holistic impact encompasses emotional well-being, social connectedness, and a resilient cognitive foundation that enriches every facet of life.

Future Cognitive Reserve: Nurturing Mental Wealth

Consistent cognitive engagement serves as an investment in future cognitive reserve. Building and maintaining cognitive reserve through intellectual pursuits may potentially provide a buffer against cognitive challenges that may arise in later life. Nurturing mental wealth becomes a forward-thinking approach to safeguarding cognitive well-being.

As we navigate the landscape of continuous cognitive engagement, we uncover a rich tapestry of benefits that extend far beyond the realm of intellectual prowess. The journey becomes a testament to the dynamic interplay between mind and experience, where the pursuit of knowledge and curiosity becomes a lifelong companion on the path to cognitive vitality.

Social Connections and Cognitive Well-being

Importance of Social Relationships

In the intricate tapestry of human experience, social relationships stand as the vibrant threads that weave together the fabric of our lives. Lets explore the multifaceted impact of relationships on our emotional well-being, mental health, and overall quality of life.

Emotional Support: The Pillars of Resilience

Social relationships serve as the pillars of emotional support, offering a foundation of resilience in the face of life's challenges. Trusted friends, family, and companions provide a safety net, creating a space where emotions can be expressed, understood, and validated. The strength of these connections becomes a buffer against the storms of life.

Mental Health and Well-being: The Social Prescription

Engaging in meaningful social relationships acts as a powerful prescription for mental health and overall well-being. Regular social interactions contribute to the release of oxytocin and serotonin—neurotransmitters associated with happiness and stress reduction. The social prescription becomes a vital component in maintaining a balanced and resilient mental landscape.

Sense of Belonging: The Community Tapestry

Social relationships weave a community tapestry that fosters a profound sense of belonging. Being part of social circles, whether family, friends, or wider communities, fulfills the innate human need for connection. The sense of belonging becomes a cornerstone in shaping identity and providing a framework for understanding one's place in the world.

Stress Reduction and Coping Mechanisms: The Shared Burden

Sharing life's burdens with others in our social network becomes a potent stress reduction and coping mechanism. Whether through shared laughter, empathetic conversations, or collaborative problem-solving, social relationships distribute the weight of challenges. The shared burden lightens individual loads and enhances the ability to navigate stressful situations.

Development of Empathy and Emotional Intelligence: The Social Skills Workshop

Interacting with diverse individuals cultivates empathy and emotional intelligence—a set of social skills crucial for navigating complex human interactions. Understanding others' perspectives, recognizing emotions, and effectively communicating feelings are honed in the social skills workshop provided by meaningful relationships.

Social Influence on Behavior: The Peer Effect

Social relationships exert a considerable influence on individual behavior. The peer effect, observed in both positive and negative contexts, showcases the impact of social circles on decision-making, habits, and lifestyle choices. Awareness of this influence underscores the importance of cultivating positive and supportive social environments.

Longevity and Health Outcomes: The Wellness Connection

Research suggests a connection between the quality of social relationships and longevity. Maintaining robust social connections has been associated with improved health outcomes, including lower rates of chronic diseases, enhanced immune function, and a higher likelihood of adopting health-promoting behaviors. The wellness connection highlights the intricate link between social bonds and overall health.

Social Support Networks in Adversity: The Safety Net

During times of adversity, social support networks become a safety net that provides comfort and assistance. Whether facing personal challenges, health crises, or major life transitions, the presence of a supportive social circle enhances coping mechanisms and contributes to resilience in navigating difficult circumstances.

Quality vs. Quantity: Nurturing Meaningful Connections

While the quantity of social relationships matters, the quality of these connections holds paramount importance. Nurturing meaningful relationships involves investing time and energy in building deep, authentic connections. Fostering quality relationships contributes to a richer emotional tapestry and a more profound impact on overall well-being.

Building and Sustaining Social Connections: The Art of Connection

Building and sustaining social connections is an art that requires intentionality, communication, and mutual investment. Engaging in shared activities, active listening, and expressing genuine care contribute to the art of connection. The deliberate cultivation of social relationships enhances the richness of life's experiences.

As we navigate the importance of social relationships, we unravel a tapestry of emotional resilience, mental well-being, and a sense of belonging. The profound impact of meaningful connections underscores the integral role that social relationships play in shaping the human experience and fostering a life of depth, meaning, and interconnectedness.

Building and Maintaining Social Connections

he dynamic landscape of human relationships, the ability to build and maintain social connections is a skill set that enriches the tapestry of our lives. This chapter explores the art and strategies of cultivating meaningful connections, delving into the nuances of initiating, nurturing, and sustaining relationships that contribute to our emotional well-being and overall quality of life.

Initiating Social Connections: The First Brushstroke

Initiating social connections is akin to creating the first brushstroke on the canvas of friendship. Small gestures, such as initiating conversations, expressing genuine interest, and extending invitations, serve as the initial strokes that lay the foundation for meaningful connections. The art of initiation involves stepping into the canvas of potential relationships with openness and authenticity.

Active Listening and Empathy: The Heart of Connection

Active listening and empathy form the heart of connection. The art of truly hearing others, understanding their perspectives, and responding with empathy fosters a deep sense of connection. Engaging in meaningful conversations, asking open-ended questions, and validating others' experiences contribute to the art of building rapport and establishing bonds.

Shared Activities and Interests: The Canvas of Commonality

Shared activities and interests become the canvas of commonality, providing a backdrop for the development of connections. Engaging in activities that resonate with personal interests creates natural opportunities for connection. Whether through shared hobbies, group activities, or collaborative projects, the canvas of commonality becomes a vibrant space for relationship building.

Communication Skills: The Brushstrokes of Connection

Effective communication skills are the brushstrokes that define the quality of connections. Clear and respectful communication, the ability to express oneself authentically, and being receptive to others' perspectives contribute to the art of connection. The nuances of verbal and nonverbal communication become essential elements in the creation of meaningful relationships.

Building Trust: The Foundation of Connection

Trust serves as the foundation of meaningful connections. Consistency, reliability, and authenticity contribute to the establishment of trust in relationships. The art of building trust involves being dependable, maintaining confidentiality, and demonstrating integrity. Trust becomes the cornerstone upon which lasting connections are built.

Navigating Social Dynamics: The Art of Adaptation

Understanding and navigating social dynamics is an aspect of the art of connection. Recognizing the diversity of personalities, adapting communication styles, and being attuned to social cues contribute to successful relationship building. The art of adaptation involves a flexible and open-minded approach to navigating the intricacies of social interactions.

Cultivating Friendships: The Garden of Connection

Friendships require cultivation, much like tending to a garden. Regular nurturing, checking in, and being present in friends' lives contribute to the growth of connections. Celebrating successes, providing support during challenges, and being a consistent presence in the garden of connection foster the depth and resilience of friendships.

Overcoming Barriers: The Art of Connection Resilience

Overcoming barriers is an inherent aspect of the art of connection resilience. Challenges such as misunderstandings, conflicts, or periods of distance are natural in relationships. The ability to navigate these challenges, engage in open communication, and seek resolution contributes to the resilience of connections.

Sustaining Long-Distance Connections: The Thread Across

Distances

In our interconnected world, sustaining long-distance connections is an art that transcends physical boundaries. Utilizing technology for regular communication, planning visits, and finding creative ways to stay connected become essential brushstrokes in maintaining relationships across distances. The thread across distances becomes a testament to the enduring nature of meaningful connections.

Mindful Social Media Engagement: The Digital Palette

In the age of digital connectivity, mindful social media engagement becomes part of the art of connection. Balancing online interactions with in-person connections, using social media to enhance, not replace, face-to-face relationships, and being intentional in digital communication contribute to a balanced and healthy digital palette of connections.

Celebrating Diversity: The Mosaic of Relationships

Celebrating diversity in relationships enriches the mosaic of connection. Embracing relationships with individuals from diverse backgrounds, cultures, and perspectives broadens our understanding of the world. The art of connection involves appreciating the unique qualities that each person brings to the mosaic of relationships.

As we explore the art of building and maintaining social connections, we embark on a journey where every interaction becomes a brushstroke, contributing to the masterpiece of our social landscape. The nuances of initiation, communication, trust-building, and adaptation shape the canvas of connection, creating a vibrant tapestry that adds depth, color, and meaning to the human experience.

Community Involvement and Its Impact

Within the complex network of human relationships, active participation in the community stands out as a formidable influence, molding not only our immediate environment but also fostering enduring effects on personal welfare. This section delves into the importance of engaging with one's community, unveiling the diverse advantages it bestows upon individual development, social connections, and the broader tapestry of society.

Active Participation: The Catalyst for Change

Active participation in the community acts as a catalyst for positive change. Whether through volunteering, joining community initiatives, or contributing skills, active involvement empowers individuals to play an active role in shaping the environment they inhabit. The act of participation becomes a dynamic force in driving community growth and improvement.

Sense of Belonging: The Heartbeat of Community

Community involvement fosters a profound sense of belonging. Engaging with fellow community members in shared activities, events, or projects creates a collective identity. The heartbeat of community pulses through the connections formed, providing individuals with a deeper connection to the place they call home.

Building Social Networks: The Community Tapestry

Participating in community activities weaves a rich tapestry of social networks. The connections formed in community involvement extend beyond immediate circles, creating a diverse web of relationships. Whether through collaborative projects, neighborhood events, or shared interests, the community tapestry becomes a vibrant mosaic of interconnected lives.

Personal Growth and Development: The Community Classroom

Community involvement serves as a classroom for personal growth and development. Engaging in diverse roles and responsibilities within the community provides individuals with opportunities to enhance leadership skills, communication abilities, and problem-solving capacities. The community classroom becomes a fertile ground for honing a spectrum of valuable life skills.

Civic Responsibility: The Cornerstone of Democracy

Active community involvement instills a sense of civic responsibility—a cornerstone of a thriving democracy. Understanding one's role in contributing to the common good, participating in civic processes, and advocating for positive change become integral aspects of responsible citizenship. The sense of civic duty becomes the driving force behind community engagement.

Enhanced Well-being: The Community Wellness Effect

Research suggests a positive correlation between community involvement and enhanced well-being. The sense of purpose derived from contributing to something larger than oneself, the social connections formed, and the feeling of making a difference contribute to overall life satisfaction. The community wellness effect becomes a testament to the holistic impact of active engagement.

Youth Empowerment: Nurturing Future Leaders

Community involvement plays a pivotal role in nurturing future leaders. Providing young individuals with opportunities to actively contribute to their community fosters a sense of empowerment. The skills and values cultivated through early engagement become the foundation for responsible and compassionate leadership in the future.

Cultural Enrichment: Embracing Diversity

Community involvement serves as a platform for cultural enrichment. Collaborating with individuals from diverse backgrounds, participating in multicultural events, and celebrating community traditions contribute to a broader understanding and appreciation of cultural diversity. The embrace of diversity becomes a hallmark of inclusive and vibrant communities.

Resilient Communities: The Bond of Support

Communities actively engaged in collaborative endeavors tend to be more resilient in the face of challenges. The bond of support formed through community involvement becomes a crucial resource during times of adversity. Whether facing environmental concerns, economic challenges, or social issues, resilient communities draw strength from their collective efforts.

Environmental Stewardship: Caring for Our Common Home

Community involvement extends to environmental stewardship, as individuals collectively care for their common home. Participating in sustainability initiatives, conservation projects, and community clean-ups fosters a shared responsibility for the environment. The commitment to environmental well-being becomes a testament to the interconnectedness of community and the natural world.

Legacy of Positive Change: Leaving a Lasting Impact

Individuals engaged in community involvement contribute to a legacy of positive change. The impact of their collective efforts reverberates through the generations, shaping the ethos of the community. The legacy becomes a testament to the enduring power of individuals working together for the betterment of their shared spaces.

As we delve into the realm of community involvement, we discover a tapestry woven with threads of connection, personal growth, and positive transformation. The impact of active participation extends beyond individual lives, creating a vibrant and resilient community that thrives on the collaborative efforts of its members.

Managing Stress and Emotional Health

Stress and Cognitive Decline

In the demanding landscape of adulthood, where responsibilities often feel like a juggling act, stress becomes a common companion. This chapter explores the intricate relationship between stress and cognitive decline, shedding light on the physiological and cognitive consequences of navigating life under persistent stress.

The Unseen Weight of Adulting

As adults, the daily grind can be intense—juggling work commitments, family responsibilities, and personal aspirations. The weight of these demands often translates into chronic stress, a silent force that can subtly undermine cognitive functions over time.

Physiological Responses: The Body's Chemical Symphony

When stress becomes a persistent presence, our bodies orchestrate a chemical symphony. Stress hormones, such as cortisol, flood our system, gearing us up for perceived challenges. However, this heightened state, when prolonged, can have adverse effects on the brain, particularly areas crucial for memory and learning.

Cognitive Functions on the Line: Memory and Decision-Making

The intricate dance of stress hormones impacts cognitive functions, with memory and decision-making taking center stage. Chronic stress can compromise the functioning of the hippocampus, a key player in memory formation, leading to difficulties in recalling information and making sound decisions.

Professional Pressure: Stress in the Workplace

The professional realm often serves as a breeding ground for stress. Meeting deadlines, navigating office dynamics, and striving for career milestones create an environment where stress can thrive. This occupational stress, when unchecked, may contribute to cognitive decline, affecting performance and strategic thinking.

The Cognitive Toll of Burnout

In the pursuit of professional success, burnout can become a formidable adversary. The chronic state of physical and emotional exhaustion associated with burnout has cognitive repercussions. Memory lapses, reduced attention span, and impaired problem-solving abilities are often hallmarks of cognitive decline in the face of burnout.

Emotional Well-being: Stress's Ripple Effect

Beyond its impact on cognitive functions, stress casts a wide net over emotional well-being. The strain of constant stress can lead to feelings of anxiety, irritability, and even depression. The emotional toll further complicates the cognitive landscape, emphasizing the interconnected nature of mental and cognitive health.

Strategies for Stress Management: Preserving Cognitive Vitality

Recognizing the toll that chronic stress can take on cognitive health, adopting effective stress management strategies becomes paramount. Techniques such as mindfulness, regular physical activity, and cultivating a strong support network are instrumental in mitigating the cognitive decline associated with persistent stress.

Balancing Act: Navigating Responsibilities Mindfully

Achieving a balance between responsibilities and self-care is a delicate act. Prioritizing mental and cognitive well-being alongside professional and personal obligations is essential. Establishing boundaries, seeking support when needed, and practicing self-compassion contribute to a more sustainable and resilient cognitive framework.

Aging and Cognitive Resilience: The Role of Stress Management

As adults navigate the various stages of life, the cumulative impact of stress becomes a factor in cognitive resilience. Implementing stress management practices throughout adulthood may play a role in preserving cognitive function as individuals age. The proactive approach to cognitive well-being becomes an investment in long-term cognitive health.

In the intricate tapestry of adulthood, where stress is an inevitable thread, understanding its implications on cognitive health is key. By acknowledging the toll it takes and proactively managing stress, adults can cultivate a resilient cognitive foundation, ensuring the preservation of mental acuity and well-being throughout life's journey.

Mindfulness and Relaxation Techniques

t he fast-paced world of adulthood, where the demands of daily life can be relentless, exploring mindfulness and relaxation techniques becomes essential for maintaining mental and emotional well-being. This chapter delves into the transformative power of mindfulness, offering a toolkit of relaxation techniques to navigate the complexities of modern life.

The Art of Mindfulness

Mindfulness is more than a buzzword; it's a powerful practice that cultivates awareness and presence in the current moment. In a world brimming with distractions, the ability to anchor oneself in the present can be a game-changer for managing stress and promoting overall well-being.

Mindful Breathing: A Gateway to Calm

The breath is a constant companion, yet its significance often goes unnoticed. Mindful breathing, a cornerstone of mindfulness practice, involves paying attention to the breath's natural rhythm. This simple act serves as a gateway to calm, promoting relaxation and centering the mind amidst the chaos of daily life.

Body Scan Meditation: Unraveling Tension

Our bodies often bear the brunt of stress, harboring tension that goes unnoticed. Body scan meditation involves systematically directing attention to different parts of the body, unraveling tension and fostering a deep sense of relaxation. This practice enhances body-mind connection and promotes a state of tranquility.

Guided Imagery: Creating Mental Havens

The mind is a powerful landscape, and guided imagery taps into its potential for relaxation. Visualization of serene landscapes, peaceful scenes, or positive experiences serves as a mental haven. Engaging the imagination in this way can transport individuals to a state of calm, offering respite from the demands of reality.

Mindful Walking: Movement with Purpose

Incorporating mindfulness into daily activities, even something as simple as walking, can be transformative. Mindful walking involves bringing attention to each step, the sensation of movement, and the surrounding environment. This practice not only promotes relaxation but also enhances awareness of the present moment.

Progressive Muscle Relaxation: Releasing Physical Tension

Physical tension often accompanies stress, and progressive muscle relaxation provides a systematic approach to releasing it. By tensing and then gradually releasing different muscle groups, individuals can cultivate awareness of physical sensations and promote a state of deep relaxation.

Mindfulness Meditation: Cultivating Inner Stillness

Mindfulness meditation is a formal practice that involves sitting quietly and directing attention to the breath, sensations, or a focal point. This intentional focus cultivates inner stillness, allowing individuals to observe thoughts without attachment. Regular mindfulness meditation is associated with reduced stress, improved emotional regulation, and enhanced cognitive function.

Yoga and Tai Chi: Movement as Meditation

Yoga and Tai Chi combine movement with mindfulness, offering holistic practices that promote relaxation and flexibility. These mind-body disciplines involve intentional breathwork, gentle postures, and flowing movements, fostering a harmonious connection between body and mind. Incorporating yoga or Tai Chi into a routine can be a transformative step toward stress management.

Mindful Eating: Savoring the Experience

Amidst hectic schedules, meals are often rushed and mindless. Mindful eating encourages individuals to savor each bite, paying attention to flavors, textures, and the act of eating itself. This practice not only enhances the enjoyment of meals but also fosters a mindful approach to nourishment and self-care.

Journaling: Reflection for Relaxation

The act of journaling provides an outlet for self-reflection and expression. Taking time to jot down thoughts, emotions, and experiences can be a cathartic practice. Journaling fosters self-awareness, allowing individuals to process stressors and gain insights into their inner landscape.

Integrating Mindfulness into Daily Life: Sustainable Practices

The effectiveness of mindfulness and relaxation techniques lies in their integration into daily life. Rather than viewing these practices as separate from the hustle and bustle, incorporating them into routine activities creates sustainable habits. Small, consistent steps lead to lasting benefits for mental and emotional well-being.

The Mindful Pause: A Breath Amidst Chaos

In the whirlwind of daily life, the mindful pause offers a breath amidst chaos. Taking intentional breaks to practice a brief moment of mindfulness—whether through a few deep breaths, a short meditation, or a conscious pause—becomes a powerful tool for navigating stress and cultivating resilience.

Mindfulness Apps and Resources: Technology for Well-being

In the digital age, technology can serve as a supportive ally on the mindfulness journey. Numerous apps and online resources offer guided meditations, breathing exercises, and mindfulness tools. Integrating these resources into daily life provides accessible and personalized support for relaxation and well-being.

Mindfulness in Community: Shared Practices

Engaging in mindfulness practices within a community setting adds a dimension of shared experience and support. Group meditation sessions, mindfulness workshops, or joining online communities create opportunities for connection and the collective cultivation of well-being.

Mindfulness as a Lifelong Journey: The Path to Resilience

Mindfulness and relaxation techniques are not quick fixes but rather lifelong companions on the journey to resilience. Regular practice cultivates a mindset that can navigate challenges with greater ease, fostering emotional intelligence, and promoting overall mental well-being.

In the tapestry of adult life, where stress is woven into the fabric of responsibilities, mindfulness and relaxation techniques offer a sanctuary of calm. By embracing these practices, individuals can reclaim moments of tranquility, enhance their capacity to respond to life's demands, and embark on a journey of self-discovery and well-being.

Emotional Resilience and Brain Health

The intricate interplay between emotions and cognitive well-being, the concept of emotional resilience emerges as a cornerstone for maintaining a healthy and agile brain. This chapter explores the dynamic relationship between emotional resilience and brain health, unraveling the profound impact of our emotional landscape on cognitive function.

Understanding Emotional Resilience

Emotional resilience is not about suppressing emotions or avoiding difficulties; it's about navigating challenges with adaptability and bounce-back ability. This quality allows individuals to confront stressors, setbacks, and life's inevitable curveballs with a mindset that fosters growth and well-being.

The Emotional Brain: A Nexus of Experience

The brain and emotions share an intricate connection, with the limbic system playing a central role in processing emotions. Emotional experiences shape neural pathways, creating a dynamic interplay between emotional responses and cognitive function. The way we navigate and respond to emotions influences the brain's structural and functional landscape.

Impact of Chronic Stress on Emotional Resilience

Chronic stress acts as a formidable adversary to emotional resilience. Prolonged exposure to stress hormones, such as cortisol, can disrupt the intricate balance of neurotransmitters in the brain, affecting mood regulation and emotional stability. As a result, emotional resilience becomes compromised, leading to heightened vulnerability to stressors.

Neuroplasticity: The Brain's Adaptive Power

Neuroplasticity, the brain's ability to reorganize and adapt, plays a crucial role in emotional resilience. Positive experiences, coping strategies, and resilience-building activities contribute to the rewiring of neural circuits. Conversely, chronic stress and negative emotional patterns can shape the brain in ways that hinder emotional resilience and cognitive flexibility.

Emotional Resilience as a Buffer Against Cognitive Decline

Research suggests that emotional resilience serves as a protective buffer against cognitive decline. Individuals with higher emotional resilience may experience slower rates of cognitive aging and a reduced risk of developing neurodegenerative disorders. The capacity to navigate life's emotional ups and downs may contribute to the maintenance of cognitive vitality.

Mind-Body Connection: Emotional Resilience in Action

The mind-body connection becomes a tangible expression of emotional resilience. Practices such as meditation, yoga, and mindful breathing not only promote emotional well-being but also influence the brain's structure and function. These mind-body practices enhance emotional regulation, stress response modulation, and contribute to the cultivation of a resilient mindset.

Positive Psychology: Nurturing Emotional Well-being

Positive psychology emphasizes the cultivation of strengths, positive emotions, and a sense of purpose. Embracing gratitude, fostering positive relationships, and engaging in activities that bring joy contribute to emotional resilience. This intentional focus on positive aspects of life not only enhances emotional well-being but also influences the brain's neurochemistry.

Cognitive Appraisal: Shaping Emotional Responses

How we perceive and appraise situations influences emotional resilience. Cognitive appraisal, the way we interpret events, plays a pivotal role in shaping emotional responses. Adopting a mindset that views challenges as opportunities for growth, reframing negative thoughts, and cultivating self-compassion contribute to a more resilient approach to life's emotional complexities.

Social Support Networks: Pillars of Emotional Resilience

The presence of a strong social support network contributes

significantly to emotional resilience. Meaningful connections, whether with friends, family, or a community, provide a buffer against stress and enhance emotional well-being. Social support not only influences emotional resilience but also contributes to the release of neurochemicals that promote brain health.

Emotional Intelligence: A Catalyst for Resilience

Emotional intelligence, encompassing self-awareness, self-regulation, empathy, and interpersonal skills, serves as a catalyst for emotional resilience. Cultivating emotional intelligence enhances the ability to navigate emotions effectively, fostering a balanced and adaptive response to life's challenges.

Resilience-Building Strategies: A Holistic Approach

Building emotional resilience involves a holistic approach that integrates various strategies. Mindfulness practices, positive psychology interventions, cognitive-behavioral techniques, and nurturing social connections collectively contribute to a resilient mindset. This multifaceted approach enhances emotional well-being and fortifies the brain against the detrimental effects of chronic stress.

A Lifelong Journey: Nurturing Brain Health Through Resilience

Embracing emotional resilience as a lifelong journey becomes a proactive investment in brain health. As individuals cultivate the ability to bounce back from adversity, adapt to changing circumstances, and foster positive emotional states, they contribute to the well-being of their brains. The dynamic interplay between emotional resilience and brain health underscores the profound influence of our emotional landscape on cognitive function.

Embracing Emotional Resilience for a Vibrant Brain

In the intricate tapestry of brain health, emotional resilience emerges as a vibrant thread that weaves through every emotional experience. Nurturing this resilience not only fosters well-being in the face of life's challenges but also becomes a cornerstone for maintaining cognitive vitality. As we navigate the complexities of our emotional landscape, let us embark on a journey of resilience—a journey that not only fortifies our minds but enriches the very fabric of our lives.

Medical Interventions and Treatments

Medications for Cognitive Decline

C ognitive decline is a complex challenge, and exploring medications and proven strategies is a crucial step in addressing this issue. This chapter delves into the medications available for cognitive decline, alongside evidence-based techniques and strategies that have shown efficacy in supporting cognitive function.

Understanding Medications for Cognitive Decline

Several medications are prescribed to address cognitive decline, particularly in conditions like Alzheimer's disease and other forms of dementia. It's essential to note that these medications aim to manage symptoms rather than provide a cure. Common medications include:

1. **Cholinesterase Inhibitors:**

- **Donepezil (Aricept):** This medication increases acetylcholine levels in the brain, a neurotransmitter associated with memory and learning.
- **Rivastigmine (Exelon) and Galantamine (Razadyne):** These medications also boost acetylcholine levels and may

provide symptomatic relief.

1. **NMDA Receptor Antagonist:**

- **Memantine (Namenda):** This medication regulates glutamate, another neurotransmitter. It is often prescribed to manage moderate to severe Alzheimer's disease.

Proven Strategies to Support Cognitive Function

While medications can play a role in managing cognitive decline, incorporating evidence-based strategies into daily life is equally important. These strategies are not only beneficial for individuals experiencing cognitive decline but also contribute to overall brain health.

1. **Regular Physical Exercise:**

- **Proven Benefits:** Exercise enhances blood flow, promotes neuroplasticity, and stimulates the release of chemicals that support cognitive function.
- **Recommendation:** Aim for at least 150 minutes of moderate-intensity aerobic exercise per week, coupled with strength training exercises.

1. **Healthy Diet:**

- **Proven Benefits:** A nutritious diet rich in antioxidants, omega-3 fatty acids, and other essential nutrients supports brain health and may reduce the risk of cognitive decline.
- **Recommendation:** Emphasize a Mediterranean-style diet, including fruits, vegetables, whole grains, fish, and olive

oil.

1. **Cognitive Stimulation:**

- **Proven Benefits:** Engaging in mentally stimulating activities builds cognitive reserve and promotes brain health.
- **Recommendation:** Stay mentally active through activities like puzzles, games, reading, learning new skills, and engaging in hobbies.

1. **Adequate Sleep:**

- **Proven Benefits:** Quality sleep is crucial for memory consolidation, cognitive function, and overall well-being.
- **Recommendation:** Aim for 7-9 hours of sleep per night, establish a consistent sleep routine, and create a sleep-conducive environment.

1. **Stress Management:**

- **Proven Benefits:** Chronic stress negatively impacts cognitive function, and effective stress management is essential for brain health.
- **Recommendation:** Incorporate stress-reducing practices such as mindfulness, meditation, deep breathing, and relaxation techniques.

1. **Social Engagement:**

- **Proven Benefits:** Social interactions contribute to cognitive reserve and emotional well-being.

- **Recommendation:** Stay socially connected through regular interactions with friends, family, and community activities.

1. **Heart-Healthy Practices:**

- **Proven Benefits:** What's good for the heart is often good for the brain. Managing conditions like hypertension, diabetes, and high cholesterol is crucial.
- **Recommendation:** Follow heart-healthy practices, including regular medical check-ups and adherence to prescribed medications.

1. **Mental Health Support:**

- **Proven Benefits:** Addressing mental health conditions, such as depression and anxiety, is essential for overall cognitive well-being.
- **Recommendation:** Seek professional support if experiencing mental health challenges, and consider therapies that focus on cognitive and emotional aspects.

Combining Medications with Lifestyle Strategies

While medications offer symptomatic relief, combining them with lifestyle strategies can maximize their effectiveness and contribute to long-term cognitive health. A holistic approach that addresses both pharmacological and non-pharmacological aspects creates a comprehensive plan for managing cognitive decline.

The Importance of Individualized Approaches

It's crucial to recognize that the impact of medications and strategies can vary from person to person. Individualized approaches, tailored to the unique needs and circumstances of each individual, are key. Regular consultation with healthcare professionals, including physicians, neurologists, and other specialists, ensures a personalized and optimized care plan.

A Comprehensive Approach to Cognitive Health

In navigating the complexities of cognitive decline, a comprehensive approach that combines medications with evidence-based lifestyle strategies is paramount. Medications may provide symptomatic relief, but the proactive integration of lifestyle practices contributes to overall cognitive health and well-being.

Through this integrated approach, individuals can forge a path toward enhanced cognitive function, resilience, and a fuller, more enriched life.

Emerging Therapies and Research

The landscape of cognitive health is continuously evolving, and emerging therapies and research offer a glimpse into the future of addressing cognitive decline. This chapter explores promising avenues in the field, incorporating both emerging therapies and proven strategies supported by ongoing research.

1. Gene Therapy: Unlocking Genetic Potential

Current Developments: Gene therapy is at the forefront of innovative approaches to cognitive health. Researchers are exploring the potential of modifying or replacing genes associated with cognitive disorders to address underlying genetic factors.

Proven Strategies: While gene therapy is still in its early stages, adopting a lifestyle that supports overall well-being can positively influence gene expression. Regular exercise, a balanced diet, and stress management contribute to genetic factors linked to cognitive health.

**2.   Neurostimulation Techniques: Energizing Brain

Function

Current Developments: Non-invasive neurostimulation techniques, such as transcranial magnetic stimulation (TMS) and transcranial direct current stimulation (tDCS), are under investigation. These methods aim to modulate neural activity and enhance cognitive functions.

Proven Strategies: Cognitive training exercises, combined with neurostimulation, show promise. Engaging in mentally stimulating activities, such as puzzles and memory games, alongside neurostimulation, may offer synergistic benefits.

**3. Immunotherapy: Harnessing the Immune System

Current Developments: Immunotherapy approaches are being explored to target the abnormal proteins associated with cognitive disorders. Vaccines and monoclonal antibodies are under investigation to stimulate the immune system to recognize and clear these proteins.

Proven Strategies: Adopting an anti-inflammatory diet rich in antioxidants supports overall brain health. Foods high in omega-3 fatty acids, fruits, and vegetables contribute to an environment that may mitigate inflammation.

**4. Cognitive Rehabilitation: Nurturing Neuroplasticity

Current Developments: Cognitive rehabilitation programs are evolving, focusing on enhancing neuroplasticity—the brain's ability to reorganize and adapt. Tailored interventions aim to improve specific cognitive functions through targeted exercises.

Proven Strategies: Engaging in cognitive training activities, such as memory exercises, problem-solving tasks, and language games, fosters neuroplasticity. These activities can be incorporated into daily life to support cognitive function.

5. Epigenetic Interventions: Modifying Gene Expression

Current Developments: Epigenetic interventions aim to modify gene expression without altering the underlying DNA sequence. Researchers are exploring compounds that may influence epigenetic markers to promote cognitive health.

Proven Strategies: Nutrition plays a role in epigenetic modifications. Consuming foods rich in folate, B vitamins, and other micronutrients supports methylation processes, potentially influencing gene expression related to cognitive function.

6. Virtual Reality (VR) Therapy: Immersive Cognitive Training

Current Developments: Virtual reality therapy is gaining attention for its potential in cognitive training. VR environments provide immersive experiences, allowing individuals to engage in tasks that stimulate various cognitive functions.

Proven Strategies: Cognitive training apps and games, even without VR technology, offer effective ways to engage the brain. Regular use of these tools, focusing on memory, attention, and problem-solving, can contribute to cognitive resilience.

7. Lifestyle Modification Programs: Comprehensive Approaches

Current Developments: Comprehensive lifestyle modification programs combine various interventions, including diet, exercise, cognitive training, and stress management. These programs aim to address multiple factors influencing cognitive health.

Proven Strategies: Adopting a holistic approach to lifestyle modification has proven benefits. Programs that encompass physical activity, cognitive stimulation, social engagement, and a healthy diet contribute to overall cognitive well-being.

Integrating Innovation with Proven Practices

Individuals can actively contribute to their cognitive well-being by adopting a lifestyle that incorporates physical activity, cognitive engagement, social connections, and a nutritious diet. Remaining informed about emerging therapies and participating in research studies when possible further contributes to the collective effort to advance our understanding and treatment of cognitive decline.

In this dynamic landscape, the synergy between innovation and established practices offers hope for a future where cognitive health is not only understood but actively nurtured. As we continue to unravel the mysteries of the brain, let us embark on a journey that embraces both the forefront of scientific progress and the wisdom of time-tested strategies for a resilient and vibrant cognitive life.

Challenges and Hopes in Medical Approaches

T hough battling daunting challenges, the pursuit of medical interventions for cognitive decline ignites hope with promising breakthroughs.

Challenges in Medical Approaches to Cognitive Decline

1. **Complexity of the Brain:

- **Challenge:** The intricacies of the human brain pose a formidable challenge. Its complexity and the unique nature of cognitive disorders make understanding and treating them a complex endeavor.
- **Hopeful Outlook:** Advancements in neuroimaging and molecular biology contribute to a deeper understanding of brain function. This evolving knowledge is a crucial step toward developing targeted and effective treatments.

1. **Individual Variability:

- **Challenge:** Individuals exhibit diverse responses to medical interventions, leading to variability in treatment outcomes. What works for one person may not yield the same results for another.

- **Hopeful Outlook:** Personalized medicine is gaining traction, aiming to tailor treatments based on an individual's genetic makeup, lifestyle, and specific cognitive profile. This approach holds promise for more effective and personalized interventions.

1. **Limited Treatment Efficacy:**

- **Challenge:** Some medications and interventions show limited efficacy in slowing or halting cognitive decline. The search for treatments that go beyond symptom management remains a challenge.
- **Hopeful Outlook:** Ongoing research explores innovative therapies targeting different aspects of cognitive disorders. Combining treatments and addressing multiple pathways may hold the key to more impactful interventions.

1. **Late-Stage Intervention:**

- **Challenge:** Many interventions are initiated in the later stages of cognitive decline when significant damage has already occurred. Early detection and intervention remain critical challenges.
- **Hopeful Outlook:** Advances in biomarker research and digital health technologies offer opportunities for early detection. Promoting awareness and routine cognitive assessments contribute to early intervention strategies.

Hopes and Strategies in Medical Approaches

1. **Precision Medicine:**

- **Hope:** Precision medicine, tailoring treatments based on individual characteristics, offers a promising avenue. Genetic profiling and comprehensive assessments can guide personalized interventions.
- **Strategy:** Collaborate with healthcare providers who embrace precision medicine principles, ensuring a thorough understanding of individual needs and characteristics.

1. **Innovative Clinical Trials:**

- **Hope:** Ongoing and upcoming clinical trials investigate novel therapeutic approaches. Participation in clinical trials contributes to advancing medical knowledge and potential breakthroughs.
- **Strategy:** Stay informed about clinical trials related to cognitive decline. Engaging with healthcare professionals and research institutions provides opportunities for involvement.

1. **Integrated Care Models:**

- **Hope:** Comprehensive and integrated care models, addressing both medical and lifestyle factors, show promise in managing cognitive decline.
- **Strategy:** Seek healthcare providers who adopt a holistic approach to cognitive health. Comprehensive care plans that encompass medications, lifestyle modifications, and

support networks enhance overall well-being.

1. **Digital Health Solutions:**

- **Hope:** Digital health technologies offer tools for remote monitoring, early detection, and personalized interventions. Wearable devices and apps contribute to proactive cognitive health management.
- **Strategy:** Embrace digital health solutions that align with individual preferences and needs. Regular use of cognitive training apps and monitoring tools enhances proactive management.

1. **Collaboration Across Disciplines:**

- **Hope:** Collaborative efforts between neurology, psychiatry, geriatrics, and other disciplines contribute to a more nuanced understanding of cognitive decline.
- **Strategy:** Seek healthcare providers who collaborate across disciplines, ensuring a comprehensive and collaborative approach to cognitive health.

1. **Patient and Caregiver Education:**

- **Hope:** Education empowers patients and caregivers to actively participate in cognitive health management. Informed individuals can advocate for themselves and make informed decisions.
- **Strategy:** Engage in ongoing education about cognitive health. Attend workshops, read reputable sources, and participate in support groups to enhance understanding

and coping strategies.

Navigating the Journey with Resilience and Hope

As individuals and communities navigate the journey of cognitive health, a resilient approach involves staying informed, actively participating in one's care, and embracing a comprehensive view of well-being. By understanding the challenges and fostering hope through emerging medical approaches, we pave the way for a future where cognitive decline is met with effective, personalized, and compassionate interventions.

Caregiving for Individuals with Dementia

Understanding the Caregiver Role

Though demanding and intricate, caregiving for someone with cognitive decline offers profound rewards. This guide unpacks the responsibilities, emotional impact, and strategies to navigate this crucial role with compassion and resilience.

<u>**Understanding the Caregiver's Responsibilities**</u>

1. **Physical Assistance:**

- *Responsibility:* Caregivers often provide physical support, assisting with daily activities such as dressing, grooming, and mobility.
- *Strategy:* Implement adaptive devices and modifications to the living environment to enhance the individual's independence.

1. **Medication Management:**

- *Responsibility:* Caregivers play a crucial role in ensuring medication adherence and managing treatment plans.
- *Strategy:* Develop a medication schedule, use pill organizers,

and maintain open communication with healthcare professionals regarding any concerns or changes.

1. **Emotional Support:**

- *Responsibility:* Caregivers offer emotional support, addressing the emotional challenges and stressors experienced by individuals with cognitive decline.
- *Strategy:* Foster open communication, actively listen, and seek emotional support for yourself through support groups or counseling.

1. **Safety and Supervision:**

- *Responsibility:* Providing a safe environment and constant supervision to prevent accidents or wandering is a vital caregiver responsibility.
- *Strategy:* Implement safety measures such as securing the living space, installing alarms, and ensuring continuous supervision, especially in high-risk situations.

1. **Advocacy and Communication:**

- *Responsibility:* Caregivers serve as advocates, communicating with healthcare professionals, coordinating care, and ensuring the individual's needs are met.
- *Strategy:* Maintain a detailed record of medical history, attend medical appointments, and actively communicate concerns or changes in the individual's condition.

The Emotional Impact on Caregivers

1. **Stress and Burnout:**

- *Impact:* The demands of caregiving can lead to chronic stress and burnout.
- *Strategy:* Prioritize self-care, set boundaries, and seek respite care to recharge and prevent burnout.

1. **Guilt and Emotional Strain:**

- *Impact:* Caregivers may experience guilt, feeling overwhelmed by the emotional strain of caregiving responsibilities.
- *Strategy:* Acknowledge and validate your emotions, seek support from others, and consider counseling to navigate complex feelings.

1. **Loss and Grief:**

- *Impact:* Witnessing cognitive decline involves a sense of loss and grief for both the individual and the caregiver.
- *Strategy:* Embrace support groups or counseling to navigate the grieving process and find healthy outlets for expressing emotions.

1. **Isolation:**

- *Impact:* Caregivers may feel isolated as their focus shifts entirely to the needs of the individual.
- *Strategy:* Cultivate a support network, stay connected with friends and family, and participate in community groups or online forums for caregivers.

Strategies for Navigating the Caregiver Role

1. Education and Information:

- *Strategy:* Invest time in understanding the specific cognitive condition, available resources, and potential challenges. Knowledge empowers caregivers to provide better care.

1. Respite Care:

- *Strategy:* Regularly schedule respite care to give caregivers time for self-care and relaxation. This could involve professional caregivers, family members, or support groups.

1. Effective Communication:

- *Strategy:* Foster open and honest communication with healthcare professionals, family members, and the individual with cognitive decline. Clear communication enhances collaboration and understanding.

1. Adaptive Coping Mechanisms:

- *Strategy:* Develop adaptive coping mechanisms to navigate stress. This could include mindfulness practices, deep breathing exercises, or engaging in activities that bring joy and relaxation.

1. Professional Support:

- *Strategy:* Seek professional support through counseling

or therapy to address the emotional impact of caregiving. Professional guidance provides a safe space to process emotions and develop coping strategies.

1. **Community Resources:**

• *Strategy:* Utilize community resources and support services. Many communities offer caregiver support groups, educational programs, and respite care services.

1. **Legal and Financial Planning:**

• *Strategy:* Address legal and financial matters early on, including power of attorney, healthcare directives, and financial planning. This proactive approach ensures clarity in decision-making.

Nurturing Compassion and Resilience

The caregiver role is both a challenging and compassionate journey. Understanding the responsibilities, acknowledging the emotional impact, and implementing effective strategies contribute to a caregiver's ability to provide optimal support. Through education, self-care, and a network of support, caregivers can navigate this role with compassion, resilience, and a profound sense of purpose.

Providing Emotional Support

Emotional support is a cornerstone in the care of individuals experiencing cognitive decline. This chapter explores the significance of emotional support, the challenges caregivers may encounter, and effective strategies to provide compassionate assistance while fostering emotional well-being.

Understanding the Emotional Landscape

Uncertainty and Fear:

- *Challenge:* Cognitive decline often brings uncertainty and fear, both for the individual and their caregivers.
- *Strategy:* Foster open communication to address fears and uncertainties. Acknowledge concerns and provide reassurance through consistent and empathetic dialogue.

Loss and Identity Shift:

- *Challenge:* Individuals with cognitive decline may experience a sense of loss and a shift in their identity.

- *Strategy:* Validate their emotions and memories, focus on preserving a sense of identity through familiar routines, and engage in activities that bring comfort.

Emotional Volatility:

- *Challenge:* Fluctuations in mood and emotional volatility can be common.
- *Strategy:* Cultivate patience, practice active listening, and acknowledge emotions without judgment. Provide a calm and supportive presence during moments of emotional distress.

<u>Effective Strategies for Emotional Support</u>

Active Listening:

- *Strategy:* Practice active listening by fully focusing on the individual's words and emotions. Validate their feelings and express empathy through your responses.

Validation of Emotions:

- *Strategy:* Acknowledge and validate the emotions expressed by the individual. Let them know it's okay to feel a range of emotions, and their feelings are understood and respected.

Reminiscence Therapy:

- *Strategy:* Engage in reminiscence therapy by encouraging the individual to share memories and stories from their past. This not only fosters a sense of identity but also provides comfort.

Creative Expression:

- *Strategy:* Encourage creative expression through art, music, or writing. These outlets offer a non-verbal way for individuals to communicate and express emotions.

Routine and Predictability:

- *Strategy:* Establish and maintain a consistent routine. Predictability can provide a sense of stability, reducing anxiety and emotional distress.

Mindfulness and Relaxation Techniques:

- *Strategy:* Introduce mindfulness and relaxation techniques, such as deep breathing exercises or guided meditation, to promote emotional well-being and reduce stress.

Engaging in Meaningful Activities:

- *Strategy:* Identify and engage in activities that bring joy and a sense of purpose. This could include hobbies, spending time outdoors, or participating in activities that align with the individual's interests.

Social Connections:

- *Strategy:* Foster social connections by maintaining relationships with friends and family. Social interactions contribute to emotional well-being and provide a supportive network.

Professional Support:

- *Strategy:* Seek professional support, such as counseling or therapy, to address emotional challenges. Professionals can provide coping strategies and a safe space for emotional expression.

Coping with Caregiver Stress

Self-Care:

- *Strategy:* Prioritize self-care to manage caregiver stress. Dedicate time for activities that bring joy, relaxation, and a sense of fulfillment.

Establishing Boundaries:

- *Strategy:* Set clear boundaries to balance caregiving responsibilities with personal needs. Understand that it's okay to seek support and take breaks when necessary.

Support Networks:

- *Strategy:* Cultivate a strong support network by connecting with other caregivers, joining support groups, and seeking assistance from friends and family.

Respite Care:

- *Strategy:* Utilize respite care services to take breaks and recharge. Respite care allows caregivers to step away temporarily while ensuring the well-being of their loved ones.

Building Emotional Resilience

Providing emotional support in the context of cognitive decline is a dynamic and evolving journey. By understanding the emotional landscape, implementing effective strategies, and prioritizing caregiver well-being, a foundation for emotional resilience is established. Nurturing emotional well-being not only enhances the quality of life for individuals with cognitive decline but also contributes to a compassionate and resilient caregiving experience.

Resources and Strategies for Caregivers

Helping someone who forgets things can be hard, but there are tricks to make it better. We'll share some ideas to make things easier for everyone!

**1. Education and Information Resources:

- **Online Platforms:** Explore reputable online platforms dedicated to cognitive health and caregiving. Websites like the Alzheimer's Association, AARP, and caregiver-specific forums offer a wealth of information, practical tips, and community support.
- **Local Workshops and Seminars:** Attend local workshops and seminars on caregiving and cognitive health. Community centers, healthcare facilities, and support organizations often host events that provide valuable insights and networking opportunities.
- **Library Resources:** Libraries offer a treasure trove of literature on caregiving, dementia, and cognitive health. Books, articles, and educational materials can enhance your understanding of the challenges and strategies associated with cognitive decline.

2. Support Groups and Networking:

- **Local Support Groups:** Join local support groups specifically tailored for caregivers. These groups provide a platform to share experiences, exchange tips, and connect with others facing similar challenges.
- **Online Communities:** Explore online communities and forums where caregivers share their journeys. Platforms like Reddit, Facebook groups, and dedicated caregiver forums offer a virtual space for support, advice, and camaraderie.
- **Professional Networks:** Connect with healthcare professionals specializing in cognitive health. Neurologists, geriatricians, and social workers can provide valuable insights, guidance, and referrals to additional resources.

3. Technological Tools and Apps:

- **Medication Management Apps:** Utilize medication management apps to organize and track medications. These apps often send reminders for medication schedules and help caregivers stay on top of complex medication regimens.
- **Cognitive Stimulation Apps:** Explore cognitive stimulation apps that offer engaging activities for individuals with cognitive decline. These apps can be beneficial in providing mental stimulation and promoting cognitive well-being.
- **Remote Monitoring Devices:** Investigate remote monitoring devices that enhance safety. These devices, such as smart home sensors and wearable technology, can alert caregivers to potential risks or emergencies.

4. Legal and Financial Planning:

- **Legal Consultation:** Consult with legal professionals to establish essential legal documents, including power of attorney and advance healthcare directives. These documents ensure clarity in decision-making and provide a legal framework for caregiving.
- **Financial Advisors:** Seek guidance from financial advisors to navigate the financial aspects of caregiving. Professionals can assist in budgeting, accessing financial assistance programs, and planning for long-term care.

5. Respite Care Services:

- **Professional Respite Care:** Engage professional respite care services to provide temporary relief for caregivers. These services allow caregivers to take breaks, attend to personal needs, and recharge.
- **Family and Friends Support:** Build a network of family and friends who can offer respite care. Establishing a schedule for loved ones to share caregiving responsibilities ensures consistent support.

6. Emotional and Mental Health Resources:

- **Counseling and Therapy:** Consider individual or family counseling to address emotional and mental health challenges. Therapists can provide coping strategies, emotional support, and a safe space for expression.
- **Mindfulness and Stress Reduction Techniques:** Practice mindfulness and stress reduction techniques to manage caregiver stress. Techniques such as meditation, deep breathing exercises, and yoga contribute to emotional well-

being.

Empowering Caregivers for Success

Navigating the challenges of caregiving requires a multifaceted approach, and accessing resources is key to success. By staying informed, building a strong support network, leveraging technological tools, and addressing legal and financial aspects, caregivers empower themselves to provide optimal care while maintaining their well-being. The journey of caregiving becomes more manageable and fulfilling when armed with knowledge, support, and effective strategies.

Building a Dementia-Preventive Lifestyle

Creating a Personalized Plan

Creating a personalized plan for cognitive well-being involves thoughtful consideration, collaboration with healthcare professionals, and a commitment to integrating lifestyle modifications. Let's explore step-by-step techniques and strategies to help individuals and caregivers develop a tailored plan that fosters cognitive health.

1. Assessment and Consultation:

- **Step 1: Initial Assessment:** Begin by seeking an initial assessment from a healthcare professional specializing in cognitive health. This may include a comprehensive evaluation of cognitive function, medical history, and lifestyle factors.
- **Step 2: Consultation with Specialists:** Engage in consultations with specialists such as neurologists, geriatricians, and nutritionists. These professionals can provide insights into specific areas of cognitive health and contribute to a holistic understanding of individual needs.

2. Identifying Personal Goals and Values:

- **Step 3: Reflect on Personal Goals:** Take time to reflect on personal goals and values. Consider what aspects of cognitive well-being are most important to you, whether it's maintaining independence, preserving memory, or sustaining emotional well-being.
- **Step 4: Set Realistic Objectives:** Establish realistic objectives aligned with your goals. Break down larger goals into achievable steps, creating a roadmap for progress.

3. Lifestyle Modification Strategies:

- **Step 5: Nutrition and Dietary Adjustments:** Work with a nutritionist to develop a customized dietary plan. Emphasize a balanced diet rich in antioxidants, omega-3 fatty acids, and nutrients known to support brain health.
- **Step 6: Physical Exercise Plan:** Collaborate with a fitness professional to create an exercise plan tailored to your fitness level and preferences. Incorporate aerobic exercises, strength training, and activities that enhance overall cardiovascular health.
- **Step 7: Cognitive Stimulation Activities:** Explore cognitive stimulation activities that align with your interests. This could include puzzles, memory games, learning a new skill, or engaging in hobbies that challenge the mind.
- **Step 8: Sleep Hygiene Practices:** Develop good sleep hygiene practices to ensure restful and rejuvenating sleep. This may involve creating a consistent sleep schedule, optimizing the sleep environment, and managing stress before bedtime.

4. Social Engagement and Emotional Well-Being:

- **Step 9: Establish Social Connections:** Actively cultivate social connections by participating in group activities, joining clubs, or attending events. Social engagement contributes to emotional well-being and provides a support network.
- **Step 10: Emotional Resilience Techniques:** Learn and practice emotional resilience techniques to navigate stress and emotional challenges. Mindfulness, meditation, and deep breathing exercises can be effective tools.

5. Regular Monitoring and Adaptation:

- **Step 11: Regular Check-Ins:** Schedule regular check-ins with healthcare professionals to monitor progress and address any changes in cognitive function. This ongoing collaboration ensures that the plan remains effective and can be adapted as needed.
- **Step 12: Adaptation and Flexibility:** Embrace adaptability and flexibility in the plan. Life circumstances, health conditions, and personal preferences may evolve, and the plan should be adjusted accordingly.

6. Incorporating Technology and Tools:

- **Step 13: Utilize Cognitive Training Apps:** Integrate cognitive training apps into your routine to provide additional stimulation. These apps offer a variety of exercises targeting memory, attention, and problem-solving skills.
- **Step 14: Wearable Technology:** Explore the use of wearable technology, such as fitness trackers or smartwatches, to monitor physical activity, sleep patterns, and overall well-being. These tools provide valuable insights for adjustments

to the plan.

****7. Building a Support Network:**

- **Step 15: Engage Family and Friends:** Share your personalized plan with family and friends, encouraging their support and involvement. A strong support network enhances motivation and accountability.
- **Step 16: Join Support Groups:** Consider joining support groups or communities focused on cognitive well-being. Connecting with others who share similar goals provides encouragement and shared experiences.

Empowering a Cognitive Health Journey

Creating a personalized plan for cognitive well-being is a dynamic and empowering process. By systematically assessing, setting goals, incorporating lifestyle modifications, monitoring progress, and building a support network, individuals can take charge of their cognitive health journey. This personalized approach not only enhances cognitive well-being but also fosters a sense of control and purpose in the pursuit of a resilient and vibrant mind.

Long-Term Strategies for Cognitive Health

Keeping your brain healthy is like taking a trip! Just like packing snacks for a long journey, we need to find tricks to keep our brains happy and strong. Prevention of Dementia, we'll learn fun ways to keep our minds sharp for years to come!

1. Holistic Lifestyle Integration:

- **Step 1: Reflect on Holistic Well-Being:** Consider cognitive health within the broader context of holistic well-being. Recognize the interconnectedness of physical, mental, and emotional aspects, and aim for a balanced and integrated approach.
- **Step 2: Comprehensive Lifestyle Adjustments:** Implement comprehensive lifestyle adjustments that address various facets of health, including nutrition, physical activity, sleep, and stress management. This holistic approach creates a foundation for long-term cognitive well-being.

2. Continual Learning and Cognitive Engagement:

- **Step 3: Embrace Lifelong Learning:** Cultivate a mindset of lifelong learning. Engage in activities that challenge the mind, such as learning a new language, taking up a musical instrument, or exploring diverse subjects of interest.
- **Step 4: Varied Cognitive Stimulation:** Diversify cognitive stimulation activities to continually challenge different aspects of cognitive function. Rotate between puzzles, memory games, creative pursuits, and intellectual endeavors to keep the brain adaptable.

3. Sustainable Nutrition and Dietary Habits:

- **Step 5: Adopt a Sustainable Diet:** Focus on adopting a sustainable and long-term dietary plan. Emphasize a balanced diet that includes fruits, vegetables, whole grains, lean proteins, and healthy fats. Consider consulting a nutritionist for personalized guidance.
- **Step 6: Regular Hydration:** Prioritize regular hydration as a fundamental aspect of cognitive health. Ensure an adequate intake of water to support overall well-being, including optimal brain function.

4. Routine Physical Exercise:

- **Step 7: Establish a Regular Exercise Routine:** Establish a regular exercise routine that aligns with your preferences and fitness level. Incorporate a mix of aerobic exercises, strength training, and flexibility exercises for sustained physical and cognitive benefits.
- **Step 8: Consistency is Key:** Emphasize consistency in physical activity. Regular, moderate exercise over the

long term contributes to improved blood flow, reduced inflammation, and enhanced neuroplasticity.

5. Prioritizing Quality Sleep:

- **Step 9: Prioritize Sleep Hygiene:** Maintain consistent sleep hygiene practices. Create a conducive sleep environment, establish a regular sleep schedule, and practice relaxation techniques to promote quality and restorative sleep.
- **Step 10: Address Sleep Disorders:** If sleep disorders arise, address them promptly. Consult with healthcare professionals to identify and manage conditions such as insomnia or sleep apnea, which can impact cognitive health.

6. Mindfulness and Stress Reduction:

- **Step 11: Integrate Mindfulness Practices:** Integrate mindfulness practices into daily life. Incorporate meditation, deep breathing exercises, or mindfulness-based activities to manage stress and promote emotional resilience.
- **Step 12: Identify Stress Triggers:** Identify and address stress triggers proactively. Develop coping mechanisms to navigate stressors, and seek support from healthcare professionals or counselors when needed.

7. Regular Health Check-Ups:

- **Step 13: Schedule Routine Health Check-Ups:** Prioritize routine health check-ups with healthcare professionals. Regular assessments contribute to early detection and management of potential health issues that may impact cognitive health.

- **Step 14: Cognitive Health Screenings:** Include cognitive health screenings as part of routine check-ups, especially as you age. Early identification of cognitive changes allows for proactive interventions.

8. Social Connections and Emotional Well-Being:

- **Step 15: Cultivate Meaningful Social Connections:** Foster and cultivate meaningful social connections. Regular interactions with friends, family, and community contribute to emotional well-being and provide a support network.
- **Step 16: Engage in Emotional Resilience Practices:** Actively engage in practices that enhance emotional resilience. This may involve participating in activities that bring joy, seeking professional support, and maintaining a positive outlook.

Sustaining Cognitive Vitality Over Time

Long-term cognitive health is a dynamic journey that requires ongoing commitment and adaptability. By embracing holistic lifestyle integration, continual learning, sustainable habits, and regular health monitoring, individuals can sustain cognitive vitality over the years. The synergy of these strategies not only supports cognitive health but also contributes to overall well-being, empowering individuals to lead fulfilling lives with resilient and vibrant minds.

Inspiring Stories of Successful Prevention

I nspiring stories of successful prevention provide invaluable insights into the real-world application of strategies and the transformative impact on individuals' lives. Let's highlight these narratives, offering a glimpse into the triumphs achieved through step-by-step techniques and enduring strategies.

1. Jane's Journey to Lifelong Learning:

Meet Jane, a spirited woman in her 60s who approached her retirement as an opportunity for growth. Jane's commitment to lifelong learning became her key to cognitive vitality. After enrolling in community college courses and attending diverse workshops, she expanded her intellectual horizons. Jane's journey exemplifies the power of embracing continual learning to foster cognitive resilience and adaptability.

2. Tom's Holistic Lifestyle Integration:

Tom, in his 70s, decided to take a comprehensive approach to cognitive well-being. Recognizing the interconnectedness of lifestyle factors, Tom overhauled his diet and incorporated brain-boosting foods. Regular exercise, encompassing both aerobic and strength training, became a non-negotiable part of his routine. By prioritizing quality sleep and embracing holistic lifestyle adjustments, Tom experienced enhanced cognitive function and overall vitality.

3. Maria's Mindfulness and Stress Management:

Maria, a professional in her 50s, discovered the transformative power of mindfulness and stress management. Introducing meditation, mindful breathing exercises, and yoga into her daily routine, Maria found a sanctuary for emotional resilience. Through these practices, she not only mitigated stress but also cultivated a mindset that contributed to sustained cognitive well-being.

4. Richard's Social Connection and Emotional Resilience:

Richard, an octogenarian, attributed his cognitive vibrancy to the richness of social connections. Actively participating in community events, maintaining close relationships, and engaging with clubs aligned with his interests became his fountain of youth. Richard's story illuminates the impact of social connection on emotional resilience, showcasing how a vibrant social life can be a powerful shield against cognitive decline.

5. Sarah's Cognitive Stimulation through Hobbies:

Sarah, a woman in her 60s, discovered the joy of cognitive stimulation through her hobbies. As an avid gardener and painter, Sarah immersed herself in activities that challenged her mind. The intricate planning of her garden and the creativity involved in painting provided continuous mental stimulation. Sarah's story underscores the importance of incorporating hobbies that bring joy and engage the mind as a strategy for cognitive well-being.

6. James' Commitment to Physical Fitness:

James, a retiree in his late 60s, made physical fitness a cornerstone of his cognitive health journey. Regular exercise, including brisk walks, cycling, and strength training, became James' routine. His commitment not only improved his cardiovascular health but also contributed to cognitive resilience. James' story emphasizes the profound connection between physical well-being and cognitive vitality.

Narratives of Resilience and Triumph

These real-life stories weave a tapestry of resilience and triumph in the realm of cognitive health. Each individual's journey is unique, but common threads of commitment to lifelong learning, holistic lifestyle integration, mindfulness, social connection, and physical fitness emerge. These narratives are not only stories of successful prevention but also blueprints for others seeking to embark on their cognitive health journeys.

As we celebrate these inspiring tales, let them serve as beacons of hope and guidance. By learning from those who have walked the path of successful prevention, we gain insights into the transformative potential of simple yet powerful strategies. Through commitment, adaptability, and a holistic approach, individuals like Jane, Tom, Maria, Richard, Sarah, and James have not only preserved their cognitive well-being but also illuminated a path for others to follow in their footsteps. Their stories stand as testament to the extraordinary capacity of the human spirit to safeguard and thrive.

Conclusion

Summing Up Key Takeaways

In the journey through the pages of this book, we've embarked on a comprehensive exploration of cognitive health, aiming to equip readers with knowledge, strategies, and inspiration for the prevention of dementia and the promotion of lasting brain well-being. As we conclude, let's recap the key takeaways that encapsulate the essence of our shared exploration.

1. Lifelong Learning as a Pillar of Cognitive Vitality:

Jane's story illuminated the transformative power of continual learning. Lifelong learning is not just an academic pursuit but a dynamic approach that stimulates the mind, fosters adaptability, and contributes to cognitive resilience.

2. Holistic Lifestyle Integration for Comprehensive Well-Being:

Tom's journey underscored the importance of comprehensive lifestyle adjustments. By addressing diet, exercise, sleep, and overall well-being, individuals can create a holistic foundation that supports cognitive health and vitality.

3. Mindfulness and Stress Management as Emotional Resilience Tools:

Maria's story highlighted the significance of mindfulness and stress management in cultivating emotional resilience. These practices not only alleviate stress but also contribute to a positive mindset and sustained cognitive well-being.

4. Social Connection as a Fountain of Cognitive Youth:

Richard's vibrant social life showcased the profound impact of meaningful connections on emotional well-being. Engaging with others, participating in community activities, and nurturing relationships emerged as essential elements for maintaining cognitive vitality.

5. Cognitive Stimulation through Joyful Hobbies:

Sarah's discovery of cognitive stimulation through hobbies emphasized the importance of joy in mental engagement. Pursuing activities that bring fulfillment and challenge the mind contributes to cognitive well-being.

6. Commitment to Physical Fitness for Cognitive Resilience:

James' commitment to physical fitness reinforced the connection between physical and cognitive health. Regular exercise, tailored to individual preferences and abilities, emerges as a potent strategy for maintaining cognitive resilience.

7. Narratives of Resilience as Inspirational Guides:

The real-life stories of Jane, Tom, Maria, Richard, Sarah, and James served as beacons of inspiration. These narratives showcased that successful prevention is not a one-size-fits-all approach but a mosaic of individualized strategies, adaptability, and resilience.

In Closing: An Ongoing Journey of Cognitive Well-Being

As we close this chapter of exploration, it's crucial to recognize that the journey to cognitive well-being is ongoing. The strategies, insights, and narratives shared in this book are not a destination but stepping stones on a path of continuous discovery and empowerment.

May the wisdom gleaned from these pages serve as a compass for readers, guiding them towards a future where cognitive health is not just a goal but an integral part of a fulfilling and vibrant life. Through lifelong learning, holistic lifestyle integration, mindfulness, social connection, engaging hobbies, and physical fitness, individuals can embark on a journey of resilience and triumph, fostering a cognitive well-being that endures the tests of time.

In the spirit of these shared stories and insights, may every reader find inspiration, motivation, and empowerment to navigate their unique path toward cognitive vitality and a flourishing mind. The journey continues, and the possibilities for cognitive well-being are as boundless as the human spirit itself.

Resources and References

Recommended Books, Websites, and Organizations

In the pursuit of cognitive health and the prevention of dementia, a wealth of resources exists to guide individuals on their journey. Whether seeking in-depth knowledge, practical tips, or a supportive community, the following recommendations encompass a diverse array of books, websites, and organizations dedicated to cognitive well-being.

1. Books:

a. "The End of Alzheimer's" by Dr. Dale Bredesen

- A groundbreaking work that explores a multifaceted approach to addressing Alzheimer's disease through lifestyle modifications, nutrition, and personalized interventions.

b. "Keep Sharp: Build a Better Brain at Any Age" by Dr. Sanjay Gupta

- Dr. Gupta, a renowned neurosurgeon, offers insights and practical advice on maintaining cognitive health through lifestyle choices, nutrition, and cognitive exercises.

c. "The Brain's Way of Healing" by Dr. Norman Doidge

- Dr. Doidge delves into the remarkable capacity of the brain to heal itself and explores innovative therapies that harness neuroplasticity for cognitive well-being.

d. "The Alzheimer's Solution" by Dr. Dean Sherzai and Dr. Ayesha Sherzai

- A comprehensive guide that emphasizes lifestyle interventions, including nutrition, exercise, and mental stimulation, as a means to prevent and manage Alzheimer's disease.

2. Websites:
  a. Alzheimer's Association (alz.org)

- An authoritative resource offering a wealth of information on Alzheimer's and dementia, including educational materials, caregiver support, and the latest research updates.

b. AARP Brain Health (aarp.org/health/brain-health)

- A dedicated section by AARP focusing on brain health, providing articles, quizzes, and resources to promote cognitive well-being in aging.

c. Mayo Clinic - Healthy Lifestyle (mayoclinic.org/healthy-lifestyle)

- Mayo Clinic's comprehensive guide to healthy living includes insights into maintaining cognitive health through nutrition, exercise, and stress management.

d. Lumosity (lumosity.com)

- An online platform offering cognitive training games designed to challenge various aspects of memory, attention, and problem-solving skills.

3. Organizations:

a. Alzheimer's Foundation of America (alzfdn.org)

- A non-profit organization providing support, resources, and advocacy for individuals living with Alzheimer's and their families.

b. Brain & Behavior Research Foundation (bbrfoundation.org)

- Committed to advancing mental health research, this foundation supports groundbreaking studies that contribute to our understanding of cognitive health and mental well-being.

c. National Institute on Aging (nia.nih.gov)

- A part of the National Institutes of Health, NIA focuses on aging-related research, providing valuable information on cognitive health, Alzheimer's disease, and related topics.

d. Dementia Action Alliance (daanow.org)

- A coalition of individuals and organizations working towards creating communities where individuals with dementia can live fully engaged and respected lives.

Navigating the Wealth of Resources

As we conclude this exploration, it's essential to recognize that the landscape of cognitive health is vast and ever-evolving. The recommended books, websites, and organizations listed here serve as navigational tools, offering diverse perspectives, evidence-based insights, and support networks.

Readers are encouraged to explore these resources, engage with the communities, and continue their quest for knowledge. The journey to cognitive well-being is enriched by curiosity, adaptability, and the collective wisdom shared by experts, authors, and organizations committed to advancing our understanding of the brain and its intricate workings.

May these recommendations serve as companions on your journey, providing guidance, inspiration, and a foundation for informed decisions as you navigate the fascinating terrain of cognitive health and the prevention of dementia.

www.ingramcontent.com/pod-product-compliance
Lightning Source LLC
Chambersburg PA
CBHW050818260726
48660CB00004B/1501